Inflammation
the source of
chronic disease

BY THE SAME AUTHOR

Sleep: the elixir of life

Inflammation
the source of chronic disease

How to treat it with herbs and
natural healing

Christine Herbert
FAMH, Dip AET, BA(Hons)

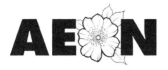

First published in 2022 by
Aeon Books
PO Box 76401
London W5 9RG

British Library Cataloguing in Publication Data
A C.I.P. for this book is available from the British Library

ISBN 13: 9781801520171

Cartoons by Lora Starling, plant drawings by Holly Gregson
Typesetting & design by Julie Bruton-Seal
Printed in Great Britain

www.aeonbooks.co.uk

Please note:
The information in this book is compiled from a blend of historical and modern
sources, from folklore and personal experience. It is not intended to replace the
professional advice and care of a qualified herbal or medical practitioner. Do not
attempt to self-diagnose or self-prescribe for serious long-term problems without first
consulting a qualified professional. Heed the cautions given, and if already taking
prescribed medicines or if you are pregnant, seek professional advice before using
herbal remedies.

Contents

continued on the next page

Preface

When looking for a suitable subject to teach to herbal students a couple of years ago I realised that understanding and treating chronic inflammation would have been a very useful subject to have studied when I had been learning some 25 years ago.

Chronic inflammation crops up with almost every person most alternative therapists see, and to consider it as an entity is a different way of looking at it – and I believe a useful one. Ignoring the name of the disease and considering the state of inflammation and where it is manifesting can be a useful way of understanding the problem.

Once I started writing lecture notes they multiplied and spread into many different avenues, so by the time I had finished I knew I had the makings of a book.

The present book owes thanks to many people, including all my herbal teachers over the years, many of whom appear here.

To my friends and colleagues Julie Bruton-Seal and Jennifer Holland, excellent therapists both who have backed me, kept me healthy and read through this book checking for errors.

To Nikki Darrell for emboldening me in the choice of subject.

To Matthew Seal for his support and editing.

To all my patients over the years for giving me the experience and learning without which I wouldn't have been able to write this.

To my publishers, Aeon, who decided that it would be worthwhile encouraging me to write.

To my good friends Lora Starling and Holly Gregson for illustrations.

And possibly most of all to my long-suffering partner Mark Naylor, who keeps me grounded, and often makes excellent practical suggestions.

The more we learn about the world, and the deeper our learning, the more conscious, specific, and articulate will be our knowledge of what we do not know, our knowledge of our ignorance
Karl Popper

Introduction

Inflammation is the underlying reason for all the major chronic diseases we see today. It is the result of many different pathological processes, which then result in one or other of:

- allergies
- arthritis
- autoimmunity
- bladder inflammation
- cancer
- cardiovascular disease
- chronic fatigue
- diabetes
- fibromyalgia
- inflammatory gut diseases
- inflammatory lung diseases
- inflammatory skin diseases
- neurodegenerative disease
- osteoporosis

and it has a big impact on mood and mental health.

There is an epidemic of chronic inflammatory diseases in the world, with incidences increasing all the time largely in response to our changing lifestyles. Instead of dying suddenly of acute infections we now die more slowly of chronic inflammatory diseases.

There are many factors that interact to determine chronic inflammatory disease. Our genes determine our individual strengths and weaknesses, but epigenetic factors control how our genes express themselves, and the way we live our life will determine this. Variable factors include diet, the environment in which we live, the health of our gut microbiome, the health of our digestive systems and of our immune system. Most of these variable factors are under our control and can be improved. Some of the methods of doing this will be found here.

This book is about chronic inflammation – the inflammation that doesn't have a useful or positive outcome in the body. Acute inflammation, with redness, swelling and heat that follows injury, is an important part of healing from an injury and needs to be allowed to proceed. The word inflammation derives from *inflamm*, to set on fire.

It is not holistic simply to stop an inflammatory response because inflammation is a result of and not a cause of disease. Inflammation is simply the body's way of defending itself against attack. This is where we have to play detective and determine the cause of the inflammation, then we can actually treat it. Anti-inflammatory medication may appear to help at first but it then becomes part of the problem if used long term.

There is further description of all the herbs mentioned together with a glossary of herbal actions in chapter 9, the materia medica.

1
What is inflammation? Acute and chronic inflammation

Everyone knows that inflammation is the combination of redness, heat and swelling that occurs after an injury or irritation of some kind to the body. It is the protective reaction of the immune system. It can be annoying, it can be extremely painful, but it is part of the healing process of the body. As such, it is an important process that must be seen through to resolution. When resolution is reached the body then produces anti-inflammatory chemicals to stop inflammation.

This should result in a return to good function and health, and end the inflammatory process. However if the cause of acute inflammation is continuous, for example untreated infection, inflammatory food and drink, or continued exposure to allergens or toxins, this becomes a chronic process that continues far longer than it should do, and causes tissue damage and malfunction and eventually chronic disease. Simply using anti-inflammatory medication to suppress the symptoms will not resolve the problem and will create new issues owing to side effects.

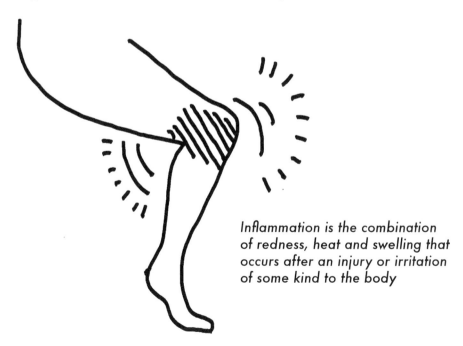

Inflammation is the combination of redness, heat and swelling that occurs after an injury or irritation of some kind to the body

Chronic inflammation is the underlying cause of most of the chronic diseases seen today:

- allergies
- arthritis
- autoimmunity
- bladder inflammation
- cancer
- cardiovascular disease
- chronic fatigue
- diabetes
- fibromyalgia
- inflammatory gut diseases
- inflammatory lung diseases
- inflammatory skin diseases
- neurodegenerative disease
- osteoporosis

and it has a big impact on mood and mental health.

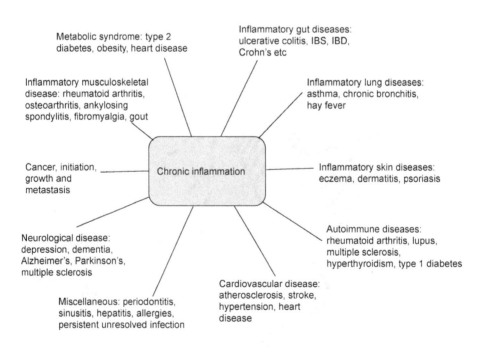

Acute inflammation is part of the body's defence mechanism. It is very important and is healing, but when it becomes chronic then the problems start. It is perfectly possible to manage acute inflammation without stopping it resolving, but the most important issue is to determine the cause of inflammation or irritation and deal with it. No amount of herbs or drugs can help if the cause is not removed.

How to treat *acute* inflammation so it resolves properly

Once the cause of inflammation – infection, injury, toxicity, allergen – has been dealt with and neutralised, then it is possible to treat the inflamed tissue with herbs and natural healing to alleviate symptoms while the body sorts itself out. If symptoms are tolerable then it is often better to allow the body to do it by itself. If not tolerable then there are some strategies that can be followed.

Improving circulation to the area will always help as it will reduce swelling and pain, and transport natural healing chemicals to the site. This can be done by alternating hot and cold compresses, or hot and cold baths. It can also be done with circulatory stimulant herbs such as cayenne or ginger, for example in a massage oil or ointment for topical treatment. Exercise, if at all possible, will also increase circulation.

Fever and heat are important to resolution of inflammation – they will kill infectious agents, or provoke sweating to expel a toxin. However, a fever above 40° Centigrade becomes dangerous and may require diaphoretic herbs (herbs that induce sweating) to help move it forward. It is important to use diaphoretic herbs 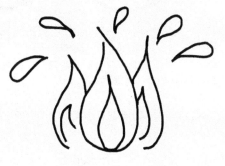 when a fever goes on for longer than two days. These include yarrow *Achillea millefolium*, ginger *Zingiber officinale*, elderflower *Sambucus nigra* and boneset *Eupatorium purpureum*.

Inflammation-mediating herbs can also be used, especially if the process is slow to resolve. These might include ginger *Zingiber officinale* or turmeric *Curcuma longa*. Using herbs to reduce inflammation is not usually directly anti-inflammatory, hence we use the term inflammation-mediating rather than anti-inflammatory. These herbs are mediating the inflammatory reaction to bring it to resolution rather than trying to stop it.

If the cause is known to be an infection – viral or bacterial – then immune herbs are really useful here. Probably the best one in an acute infection is echinacea *Echinacea purpurea* and *E. angustifolia*, although andrographis *Andrographis paniculata* is also good. Medicinal fungi, especially turkey tail *Trametes versicolor* are useful in viral infections. These should be taken in high dose for a day or two, or until symptoms are reducing.

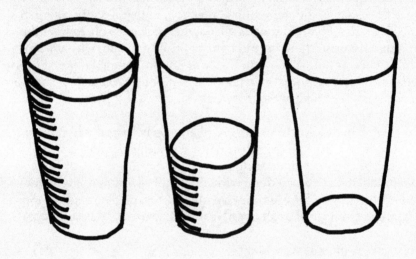

Plenty of fluids are important to prevent dehydration, and diet should be as light as possible. Rest is also important, to allow the body to get on with getting better.

Further information about all herbs can be found in chapter 9.

Inflammation is initiated by the release of chemical mediators into the spaces between tissue cells. These mediators are vasodilators, which increase blood flow to the area, creating redness and heat. The mediators also cause increased capillary permeability, which leads to swelling owing to the accumulation of fluid. Pain is due to the release of chemicals such as bradykinin and histamine that stimulate nerve endings as well as swelling that creates pressure.

The source of the mediators are damaged tissue cells, and activated cells of the immune system – phagocytes, lymphocytes, neutrophils and mast cells – that are acting to create vasodilation and increased capillary permeability by releasing mediators such as histamine, bradykinin, serotonin and prostaglandins.

Inflammation

Swelling and extra blood supply is vital to healing. The extra fluids will dilute any toxic substances and attempt to flush them out as well as supplying all the chemicals needed to fight the invasion. They will also supply blood-clotting chemicals to heal any wound, as well as being a medium for the movement of antibodies against invading pathogens.

Inflammation is regulated by prostaglandins (PG), named because they were isolated originally from the prostate gland, but now known to occur in all body tissues. These are short-lived hormones made from essential fatty acids by a long chain of reactions, the final ones being catalysed by the enzymes cyclo-oxygenase and lipoxygenase – COX and LOX.

COX converts arachidonic acid to thromboxanes (which increase blood clotting). LOX converts arachidonic acid to inflammatory leukotrienes. Some prostaglandins (PG2) are inflammatory, and some (PG1&3) are anti-inflammatory, so some are needed to start the process, and some to finish it.

Inflammation is also regulated by cytokines. These are glycoproteins that are secreted by specific cells of the immune system, which send signals to synchronise immune response and inflammation. Some cytokines are pro-inflammatory and some are anti-inflammatory – to start and then stop the inflammatory process.

Cytokine function is complex and not completely understood. Many cytokines are able to have multiple, apparently opposing functions. For example, interleukin-6 has pro-inflammatory and anti-inflammatory functions.[1] Cytokines include tumour necrosis factor TNF-alpha and interleukins IL1, 6 and 12.

The white blood cells that are attracted to the area, together with any damaged cells that need clearing up and dead bacteria, if present, will eventually result in pus formation if there are enough of them.

The white blood cells present in chronic inflammation are different from those seen in acute early inflammation. There are fewer neutrophils and more lymphocytes and macrophages in chronic inflammation. Lymphocytes are either T cells, which have cytotoxic functions, or B cells, which produce antibodies. When there are lots of B cells it suggests long-term inflammation. These new cells appear in the affected tissue and produce their inflammatory cytokines and other mediators, adding to the cycle of tissue damage and repair.

Platelets also add to the process as they aggregate in response to tissue damage, forming a clot and releasing chemokines and inflammatory mediators.

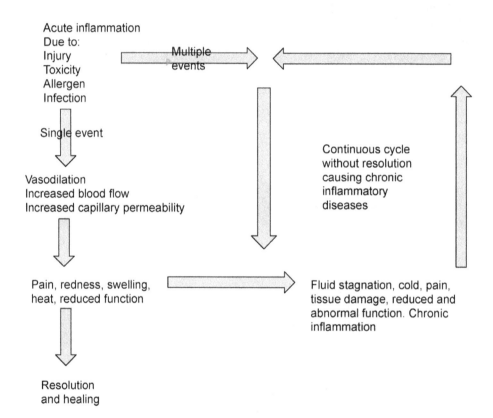

Acute inflammation
Due to:
Injury
Toxicity
Allergen
Infection

Multiple events

Single event

Vasodilation
Increased blood flow
Increased capillary permeability

Continuous cycle without resolution causing chronic inflammatory diseases

Pain, redness, swelling, heat, reduced function

Fluid stagnation, cold, pain, tissue damage, reduced and abnormal function. Chronic inflammation

Resolution and healing

Inflammation

Chronic inflammation can result from many and varied causes, including:

- A poor diet full of sugar, refined carbohydrates and trans fatty acids, mostly found in processed food, and low in vegetables, fruit and unprocessed grains, pulses, nuts and seeds.

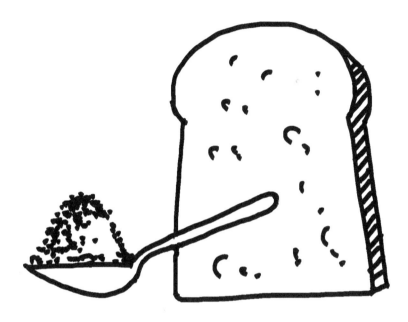

- Metabolic diseases including insulin resistance and diabetes.
- Chronic low-grade infection due to parasites, viruses, bacteria or fungi where either the immune system, or medical intervention has failed to eliminate the pathogen completely.
- Repeated episodes of acute inflammation arising from any cause.
- Autoimmune disease where the immune system constantly tries to attack body tissues – this is also a result of chronic inflammation. Examples are multiple sclerosis and rheumatoid arthritis.
- The presence of irritants in the body that cannot be removed or neutralised by the immune system. These might be foods to which there is an intolerance, irritant foods, toxic chemicals in the workplace, asbestos in the atmosphere, or moulds in the home.

There is much more about the causes of chronic inflammation in chapter 4.

Chapter summary:

- understanding acute and chronic inflammation;
- treating acute inflammation so it can resolve;
- some chemical processes involved in inflammation;
- some causes of chronic inflammation.

2
How can it be measured? Signs and symptoms showing inflammation

Inflammation can be measured by determining levels of various biomarkers in the blood. The simplest method is the erythrocyte sedimentation rate (ESR), which measures how far a column of blood will separate into red blood cells and plasma when allowed to sit vertically for one hour. When there are high levels of protein in the blood, as there are with inflammation, the ESR will be higher, but this is a non-specific and slow-changing measure of inflammation.

C-reactive protein (CRP) is found in the blood very quickly after an injury, and also can precede other evidence of inflammation. CRP is a protein made by the liver in response to inflammation, which activates the complement system to clear dead and dying tissue cells. CRP is also quick to decrease once inflammation reduces so it can be a more useful indicator of inflammation.

Homocysteine levels are less commonly tested for and are most useful as part of a cardiovascular risk assessment. Raised homocysteine levels are associated with damage to arteries and hence greater risk of cardiovascular disease.

Other, more research-oriented measures of inflammation include measurements of biomarkers such as the cytokine tumour necrosis factor (TNF-alpha), and interleukins IL-1, IL-6 or IL-8.

Another marker for increased inflammation is abnormal lipid values – chronic inflammation can increase LDL cholesterol, and decrease HDL cholesterol.[1] Anyone with high levels of LDL cholesterol is highly likely to have a chronic inflammatory process going on somewhere in their body.

Signs and symptoms of inflammation in the body will depend on the site of inflammation and how dispersed it is. However, heat, dryness, pain and lack of function are often the best signs. This can manifest as a sore, red and swollen joint, or as dry, gritty eyes, or as irritated bowels that are loose and produce many liquid or soft stools. Or it can manifest as a hot, irritable person, one who needs to drink lots of cold fluids and wears a tee shirt and shorts all year round. It can also manifest as severe fatigue and cold when it has been going for a long time – this is burnout and is far more serious as the body is by now very depleted and it will be a much harder process to get it back to health. Most chronic illness is the result of inflammation.

Inflammation case study 1

A 50-year-old male presented with a diagnosis of rheumatoid arthritis. He came to see me as soon as he had been diagnosed as he had been started on medication that he really didn't want. His medication was prednisolone, a corticosteroid, and methotrexate, an immunosuppressant, both very strong medications that suppress the inflammatory process and can have strong side effects. He knew he needed them short term but was wanting to find help so he could come off them eventually. He was also using paracetamol for pain. Leading up to this had been a long period of stress, together with a lack of care for himself with a poor diet.

Muscle testing showed dairy intolerance, but all autoimmune conditions benefit from avoiding gluten so he went on a dairy and gluten free anti-inflammatory diet.

He was advised to take vitamin D3 and good-quality fish oils; and to use turmeric *Curcuma longa* regularly, but not every day, in green smoothies and food. Ginger *Zingiber officinale* and black pepper *Piper nigrum* were also recommended to be used in his diet. All are excellent inflammation-mediating and digestive herbs, and black pepper improves absorption of turmeric.

The herbal prescription was:

- Cat's claw *Uncaria tomentosa*, an adaptogen with strong inflammation-mediating action
- Devil's claw *Harpagophytum procumbens*, an inflammation-mediating alterative
- Frankincense *Boswellia serrata*, an inflammation-mediating alterative and analgesic
- Milk thistle *Silybum marianum* for its liver- and kidney-protecting actions as well as inflammation mediation.
- He was also given *Calendula officinalis* and yarrow *Achillea millefolium* dried herbs to be made into a strong tea and used as hand baths as swollen and painful hands were one of his worst symptoms.

All these herbs were fine to be used alongside his medication, and he was able to start reducing the dose of both within about three months.

One year later he is still on methotrexate but has managed to stop prednisolone, and the dose of methotrexate is now quite low. He feels very much better and is no longer having side effects of the methotrexate now that the dose is lower. He is now looking after himself much better. He has stayed on the herbs and is likely to need them for a few months after he has stopped medication, but then hopefully will be able to continue with diet alone.

For more information about diet work and herbs, including a glossary, please see chapters 6 on diet and 9, the materia medica.

Inflammation case study 2
A 57-year-old female presented with a hyperactive thyroid gland, which was being treated with carbimazole. She had a 30-year history of asthma for which she used a salbutamol treater inhaler as needed, which was only occasionally; she had a long history of mental health illness, at times acute and needing hospitalisation, and had been taking Fluoxetine for many years. She had a history of glandular fever as a teenager and said she had never really recovered from that and often felt very fatigued. As a child she had experienced many chest infections for which she had taken numerous courses of antibiotics. She now had a more recent history of osteoarthritis in several joints, which affected her mobility. Her sleep wasn't great, waking often and also needing to get up and urinate at least once a night.

Muscle testing indicated dairy and soya intolerance.

She was put on a low-inflammation, dairy- and soya-free diet; and was recommended to take magnesium citrate to help with both sleep and the palpitations she was experiencing with her hyperthyroid condition.

A herbal formula specifically aimed at her thyroid was prescribed as a tincture:

*   Lemon balm *Melissa officinalis*
*   Gypsywort *Lycopus europaeus*
*   Motherwort *Leonurus cardiaca*

These three herbs are classically used together in hyperthyroid conditions to calm the heart and nervous system.

Another herbal formula aimed at inflammation was also made for her:

- Devil's claw *Harpagophytum procumbens*, an inflammation-mediating alterative
- Ashwagandha *Withania somnifera*, an inflammation-mediating adaptogen, helpful with sleep
- Frankincense *Boswellia serrata*, an inflammation-mediating alterative and analgesic
- Celery seed *Apium graveolens*, an inflammation-mediating alterative and digestive
- Barberry *Berberis vulgaris*, an inflammation-mediating alterative and bitter tonic

Within a few weeks her sleep was improved, she no longer needed to get up to urinate at night and she had much more energy. She stayed on the two herbal formulae for six months. By this time she had been discharged from the hospital for her thyroid condition and had been off medication for several months.

The only issue she now had was some hip pain, which occasionally affected her mobility. She thought she would like to try CBD oil as an inflammation mediator as she had heard good reports of it, and it would also be helpful as an anxiolytic. She tried it for a month and was delighted with the effects on both her hip and her anxiety, and decided this would be her preferred herbal medicine from now onwards. This was the only treatment she now needed.

For more information about diet work and herbs, including a glossary, please see chapters 6 on diet and 9, the materia medica.

Inflammation case study 3
A 34-year-old female presented with constipation and digestive problems. She had a history of severe endometriosis for which she had had a total hysterectomy and was now on hormone replacement therapy. She had a long history of severe sinusitis with antibiotic therapy and sinus surgery. Her bladder was often irritated and she had a history of multiple episodes of cystitis requiring regular antibiotics. She had difficulty going to sleep and usually awoke feeling groggy. Her back and joints were often painful and she had been diagnosed with reactive arthritis. She needed to take paracetamol daily for pain.

Although she often felt cold and shivery, 'cold to her bones', she frequently craved cold drinks and ate ice cubes. This is a classic situation of internal heat (inflammation) and poor circulation.

Muscle testing indicated nightshade and dairy intolerance, which fitted with her symptom picture and was creating a great deal of inflammation in her body.

Alongside a low-inflammation diet without dairy or nightshade family foods she was prescribed a herbal formula to improve the eliminatory and digestive function of her bowels and liver, and create a better balance of heat and cold in her body with herbs able to move body fluids as her body seemed to have become very stagnant and cold:

- Celery seed *Apium graveolens*, an inflammation-mediating alterative and digestive
- Angelica *Angelica archangelica*, an inflammation-mediating hepato-protective and digestive
- Dandelion *Taraxacum officinale*, an alterative and bitter tonic
- Yellow dock *Rumex officinale*, an alterative and lymphatic
- Barberry *Berberis vulgaris*, an alterative and bitter tonic
- She was also recommended to use ginger tea *Zingiber officinale* as an inflammation-mediating warming digestive herb.

Three weeks later her bowels were still sluggish but her digestion, bladder and sleep were all improving and she was no longer craving cold drinks and ice cubes. She needed fewer paracetamol, going two to three days at a time without any. Her sinuses felt better too.

Nightshade toxicity is very slow to improve, and it can take months to regain proper bowel function.

Six months later she came back to see me as her reactive arthritis had returned after a bout of gastroenteritis. She was craving ice cubes again and had low energy levels. She had an inflammation-mediating herbal tincture:

- Devil's claw *Harpagophytum procumbens*, an inflammation-mediating alterative
- Guduchi *Tinospora cordifolia*, primarily for joints, an inflammation-mediating alterative
- Holy basil *Ocimum sanctum*, an inflammation-mediating vulnerary and adaptogen
- Frankincense *Boswellia serrata*, an inflammation-mediating alterative and analgesic
- Gentian *Gentiana lutea*, a digestive bitter

A year later she presented with a diagnosis of reactive hypoglycaemia, which could be an early sign of diabetes so she was advised about the best diet for this.

Over the next few years she would turn up with a flare-up of her arthritis and take a herbal prescription. Unfortunately, although she always improved each time with diet and herbs, it was never a sustained improvement. She found it difficult to maintain a good diet. However, it has now been some five years since I have heard from her so it may be that she finally did beat it.

For more information about diet work and herbs, including a glossary, please see chapters 6 on diet and 9, the materia medica.

Chapter summary:

- measuring inflammation – ESR, CRP, homocysteine;
- recognising inflammation – signs and symptoms;
- case studies.

3
Inflammatory processes in the body – some of the complex networks linking them

The health of the body and the presence or absence of inflammation is dependent on the health and proper functioning of all systems and organs. Just because a knee joint is swollen and sore doesn't mean that the knee joint can be treated alone. Any body systems or organs that are malfunctioning will also need to be treated and returned to health in order to treat the knee. This is always more obvious when there is inflammation throughout the body such as in fibromyalgia or rheumatoid arthritis, but it applies to almost all chronic inflammatory processes.

The immune system
The immune system is the key to inflammation, but it doesn't work alone. It requires all body systems to play their role well in a complex interconnecting dance that, when it functions as it should, will maintain a harmony of health. It is important to understand that a strong immune system will maintain a healthy body.

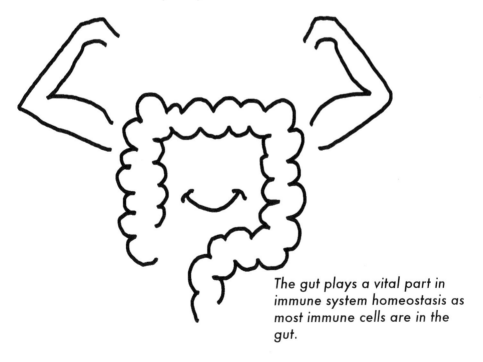

The gut plays a vital part in immune system homeostasis as most immune cells are in the gut.

The gut plays a vital part in immune system homeostasis as most immune cells are in the gut. If the gut is not healthy, the immune system won't be healthy, and there will be chronic inflammation to one extent or another. This is something that the older traditional medicine systems knew, and those who practise herbal medicine today also know. The health of the body begins in the gut.[1]

The immune system can be seen as the housekeeping system of the body. It protects us from pathogenic organisms, and removes or isolates dead or malignant body cells and foreign bodies.

Innate or non-specific immunity is the immunity we were born with, and refers to the general protective function of the immune system. It includes the barrier functions of skin and internal mucous membranes in the mouth, digestive system, lungs and urinary system. It also includes tears in the eye, and ear wax. Macrophages are also part of the innate immune system – they can eat, or phagocytose, foreign particles to render them harmless. Fever is an innate immune response, which creates a hostile environment for an invading microorganism and also stimulates the immune response.

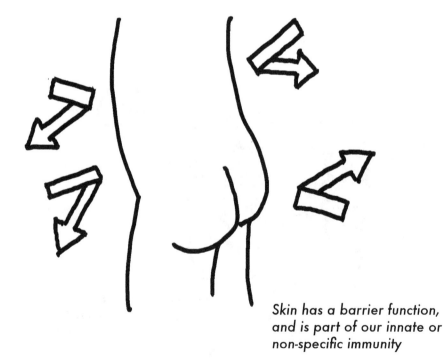

Skin has a barrier function, and is part of our innate or non-specific immunity

Inflammation

Adaptive or specific immunity develops over time in response to exposure to various antigens. It involves lymphocytes – B cells and T cells – which produce specific antibodies against the invader (B lymphocytes), and have various cytotoxic mechanisms (T lymphocytes) to clear up dead or compromised tissue cells. These cells also have an ability to remember earlier invasions, which means that future attacks are more efficiently dealt with.

A healthy immune system will recognise which cells it needs to attack, and will recognise healthy self tissue. But if it is under too much pressure, for example chronic inflammation, this is when the immune system can turn on the host body, attacking self cells and creating autoimmune disease.

Removal of dysfunctional, dead and dying tissue cells is also part of the process called autophagy (literally self-eating). This process can be seen as a spring clean of the body and may be important in protection from cancer.[2]

Autophagy involves both specific and non-specific immunity, and can be made more efficient by exercise and fasting, with the overall effect of cell regeneration and a recycling of cellular nutrients.[3]

The process of autophagy has been shown to be optimised by a diet low in refined starch and sugar and high in omega 3 fatty acids.[4,5]

How to improve the health of the immune system
Herbs and nutrition have a direct effect on the immune system, but all body systems are vital here so any attempt to improve the health of the immune system must also look at the whole.

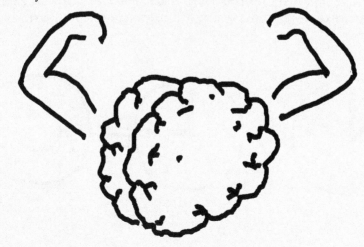

Emotional health also has an effect on the immune system, hence the field of psychoneuroimmunology. Stress or social isolation will weaken immune function, whereas a relaxed nervous system creates a strong immune system. This has been demonstrated many times in studies.[6,7,8]

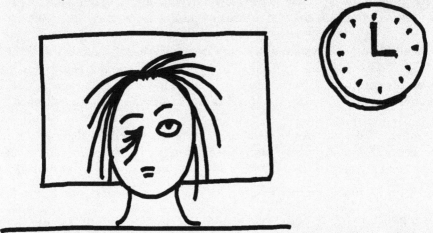

Lack of sleep is strongly linked with a weak immune system, and a much-increased risk of cancer. A study involving sleep restriction in healthy young men, where sleep was only allowed between 10 in the evening and 3 in the morning, resulted in a 70 percent reduction of natural killer cells plus reduced cellular immune response – both vital in a normal immune system, which among other things also protects us from cancer. After one night of recovery sleep only part of the immune system was returned to normal – the conclusion was that even a modest disturbance of sleep produces a reduction of natural immune response.[9]

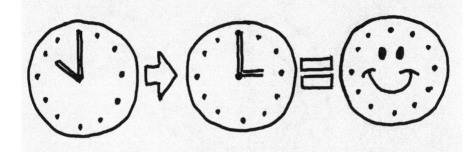

A good and varied diet is important for a healthy immune system. Particularly important vitamins and minerals include vitamins D and C, and zinc and selenium.

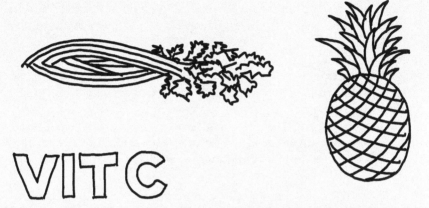

Good sources of vitamin C include most fresh fruit and vegetables; vitamin D is best obtained from sunlight exposure, or from a supplement. Food sources of vitamin D include oily fish, mushrooms and eggs. Zinc is found in red meat, shellfish, legumes, nuts and seeds. Selenium is available in brazil nuts, fish, poultry and sunflower seeds. See chapters 6 and 7 for further information about diet and supplements.

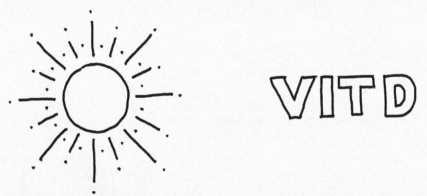

The gut microbiome needs to be healthy for a strong immune system, so fermented foods such as sauerkraut or kefir are helpful. It is important that these are unpasteurised so that the beneficial bacteria are still present.

Short-term fasting will have a stimulant effect on the immune system, as will raising the temperature of the body in a sauna or steam room. This is useful when an immediate effect is needed for an acute situation.

Herbs that have an effect on the immune system can be subdivided into those that are immune modulators or tonics – these are slower acting and can be used long term to improve immune function in those with chronic infection, autoimmune disease or lowered immunity; and herbal antimicrobials that actually attack and kill invading microorganisms.

Immune-modulating herbs include echinacea *Echinacea purpurea* and *E. angustifolia*, astragalus *Astragalus membranaceus*, marigold *Calendula officinalis*, wild indigo *Baptisia tinctoria*, Siberian ginseng *Eleutherococcus senticosus*, ginseng *Panax ginseng*, ashwagandha *Withania somnifera*, and all the medicinal fungi including *Trametes versicolor* and reishi *Ganoderma lucidum*. Many immune-modulating herbs are also adaptogens, so they will support the endocrine and nervous systems, which also support immunity.

A herb that strengthens connective tissue, and hence reinforces the barrier function of the immune system, is horsetail *Equisetum arvense*; this is a plant that is very high in silicic acid or silica, which is water soluble and required by all connective tissue.[10]

Alterative and lymphatic herbs may also have a role to play in promoting autophagy. There is a section on alterative herbs in chapter 4; lymphatic herbs might include cleavers *Galium aparine*, heartsease *Viola tricolor*, and figwort *Scrophularia nodosa*.

Herbal antimicrobials include Garlic *Allium sativum*, thyme *Thymus* spp., oregano *Origanum majorana*, sage *Salvia officinalis* and walnut *Juglans nigra*.

Further information about all herbs can be found in chapter 9, the materia medica.

The digestive system
The digestive system and inflammation are closely interlinked. In most cases of chronic inflammation the initial problem begins in the gut, generally with the diet. Either too many inflammatory foods such as sugar, trans fats or refined grains are present, or foods are eaten to which there is an intolerance, most commonly dairy or wheat. There is much more information about diet in chapter 6.

Liver health and immunity The general health of the digestive tract is dependent on the health of the gut, its microbiome and the liver. Any

Inflammation

treatment of inflammation anywhere in the body requires that the gut and the liver are both healthy and functioning well.

There is a three-way interaction between the microbiome present in the digestive system, bile acids produced by the liver, and the immune system that results in an inflammatory response, healthy or otherwise.

Bile acids are the main component of bile, produced by the liver and secreted into the small intestine via the gallbladder where its main function is to digest fats and oils from the diet. However, bile acids also have an important role to play in the inflammatory process. After they have processed fats they travel down the digestive tract where they are modified into immune- regulating molecules by gut bacteria. One type of immune-regulating molecule will activate effector helper T cells (Th17), which are pro-inflammatory, for example when there is an infection present that needs dealing with. Another type activates regulatory T cells (Tregs), which are anti-inflammatory and needed when the infecting pathogen has been killed. These cells should balance each other out to maintain good intestinal health.

Low levels of Tregs have been seen in those with inflammatory bowel disease and are linked with low bile acids.[11]

Cholestasis occurs where there is a decrease in bile flow and is associated with impaired immunity and ability to fight infection, and increased inflammation.[12]

Improving the health of the liver will improve bile acid function, and most people will benefit from improving their liver health. The functions of the liver are many, but can be simplified as follows:

- Anything that enters the body through the digestive system will eventually make its way to the liver via the bloodstream.
- The liver produces up to a litre of bile every day. This enters the small intestine via the gallbladder, which is then used to process any fats in the diet.
- The liver stores fats, and it can create fats from excess blood sugar.
- It creates cholesterol, which is used to create steroid hormones, vitamin D, the myelin sheath around neuron axons, and bile acids.
- The liver processes proteins. One of the by-products of this process is ammonia, which is toxic to the body, so the liver converts this to urea, which can then be removed from the bloodstream by the kidneys.
- The liver stores nutrients, including iron and vitamin B12.

- The liver is the organ that has to process any toxic compounds found in the body, such as alcohol, drugs and hormones, including stress hormones.
- The liver makes plasma proteins including immunoglobulins for the immune system and fibrinogen, which is involved in the clotting process.
- The liver also has an important role in keeping the blood sugar balanced as it stores glucose as glycogen until the pancreas sends a hormonal message to ask it to release glucose when blood sugar is low.

How to improve liver health
Remove anything causing harm to the liver, such as alcohol or toxic chemicals. Medication may also be causing a problem, and if this cannot be removed then work with diet to ameliorate the problem as much as possible.

Diet should be organically grown foods as much as possible in order to ensure minimal chemical residues. The website https://www.pan-uk. org/dirty-dozen/ gives an idea of how many pesticides and herbicides are used on many types of fruit and vegetables so it is possible to decide which foods should be bought as organic.

There are some foods that are good at supporting the liver. These include lemon and lime; bitter salad leaves such as dandelion, chicory and endive; dark green leafy vegetables, particularly the brassica family; and olive oil and olives. Coffee is also a useful liver herb, if not overindulged.

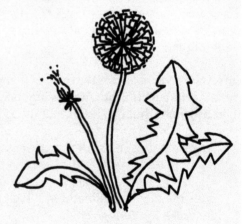

The hepatic herbs for the liver need to be chosen carefully in order to support whatever is going on. If someone has an overactive, hot liver and they are given liver-stimulant herbs they will become hot, flushed and emotional. These people need calming and cooling liver tonics. And those with a cold stagnant liver need the more stimulating liver herbs. The chart opposite is adapted from information by Michael Moore, https://www.swsbm.com/.

Inflammation

Liver herbs to improve bile production are termed cholagogues, and include those marked with an asterisk * above.

Milk thistle *Silybum marianum* is generally seen as a liver herb that can be given to either group, and is an excellent protective and restorative herb for the liver.

Further information about all herbs can be found in chapter 9, the materia medica.

Hot or overactive liver	Cold/stagnant/deficient liver
Signs and symptoms: Anabolic body state Weight gain Moist ,oily skin, often skin rashes Likes fatty and protein foods Seldom has allergies Can have low energy Hot flushes, general heat Hypertension, high blood lipids	Signs and symptoms: Catabolic body state Weight loss Dry skin Dislikes rich fatty foods Overeats carbohydrates and sweets Has blood sugar swings Prone to allergies High energy, sometimes hyperactive Can have a history of alcohol or drug use
Needs liver cooling and/or calming herbs: Agrimony *Agrimonia eupatoria* Burdock *Arctium lappa* Chamomile *Matricaria chamomilla* Dandelion *Taraxacum officinale** Rosemary *Salvia rosmarinus** Skullcap *Scutellaria lateriflora* Turmeric *Curcuma longa** Vervain *Verbena officinalis** Yarrow *Achillea millefolium*	Needs liver heating and/or stimulating herbs: Angelica *Angelica archangelica* Artichoke *Cynara scolymus** Barberry *Berberis vulgaris** Blessed thistle *Carbenia benedicta* Fringe tree *Chionanthus virginicus** Marigold *Calendula officinalis* Gentian *Gentiana lutea** Milk thistle *Silybum marianum** Mugwort *Artemisia vulgaris** Yellow dock *Rumex crispus**

Gut health The lining of the gut wall from mouth to anus is made up of many layers. The inner layer is the mucosa, in which there are mucus-secreting cells and epithelial cells. This lining is permeable but only very selectively, allowing a few small molecules to pass through once they have been digested and made safe to enter the bloodstream. The body secretes a protein called zonulin that increases intestinal permeability because some-times this is required, but this is a controlled and immediately reversible permeability. Zonulin is also secreted when there is inflammation in the gut from food sensitivities, diet, infections and so on.

When this wall is subjected to prolonged inflammatory damage, the tight junctions between cells can widen, allowing larger molecules to pass through. This then creates more inflammation owing to the activation of the immune system, and more food sensitivities. So food sensitivities are a cause of, and a result of, increased intestinal permeability.

This increased intestinal permeability is termed leaky gut and is a major player in the whole chronic inflammation process. It may also be a key process in the development of autoimmune disease.[13]

When the gut lining becomes less efficient, and the digestive secretions of the stomach decrease owing to poor health or aging, the ability of the

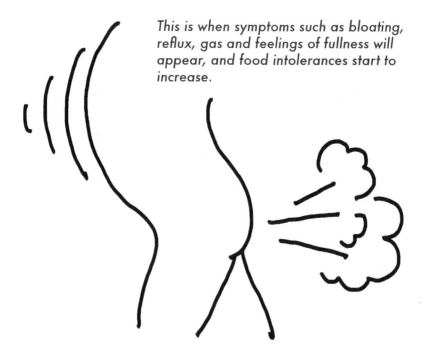

This is when symptoms such as bloating, reflux, gas and feelings of fullness will appear, and food intolerances start to increase.

Inflammation

digestive tract to actually digest food and obtain nutrients will decrease. This is when symptoms such as bloating, reflux, gas and feelings of fullness will appear, and food intolerances start to increase. These symptoms may also be related to eating the wrong foods, but often they are an indication that digestive capability has been compromised. This will have an impact on the microbiome, on the liver and on nutrient availability for the immune system. All of these factors have an impact on overall inflammation in the body. Sometimes this can be due to reduced stomach acid, which can be tested for by taking a hydrochloric acid supplement (please don't take hydrochloric acid any other way as it could cause severe burns). If the supplement creates a slight burning or reflux reaction then low stomach acid is not a problem, but if there are no symptoms it may be worth trying as a supplement.

Bacterial endotoxin is a lipopolysaccharide (LPS) found in the cell walls of gram negative bacteria, which are found in large numbers in the gut, the gums and other tissue when there is bacterial infection or dysbiosis. When they remain in the intestines they don't cause a problem, but when the bacteria die off and there is a degree of gut leakiness, then the released LPS can move through the intestinal wall and into the bloodstream where they will initiate inflammation. There is evidence to show that this process is important in the development of inflammation linked with obesity and diabetes, and may be a major cause overall of chronic inflammation,[14] and also of brain microglial activation that promotes neurodegeneration of the brain.[15]

A diet high in trans fats, or constant snacking can also cause a dysbiosis that increases LPS production,[16] and a diet high in fructose causes LPS-induced inflammation.[17] It has been shown that celery *Apium graveolens* contains aglycones, which show potent inhibitory activity against LPS-induced nitric oxide production in macrophages.[18]

Cardamom significantly decreases secretion of inflammatory mediators secreted by lipopolysaccharide-stimulated macrophages.[19]

How to improve gut health

Leaky gut and digestive ability are closely linked; once the correct diet for the individual has been found the rest will follow. Healing a leaky gut must commence with a good diet, with no inflammatory foods. See chapter 6.

Removing processed foods and replacing them with healthy food can turn around an inflamed digestive system within a couple of months. Bone broths, when long-cooked, release collagen peptides that support the repair of the intestinal wall.

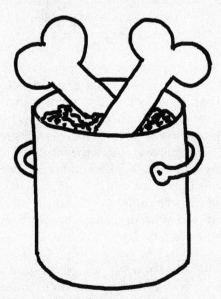

Bone broth can support the repair of the intestinal wall

Gum acacia is another supplement that appears to be able to heal damaged tissue, possibly by supporting that part of the microbiome that improves tight junctions in the intestinal lining.[20] Herbs can help to repair the gut wall, and those containing mucilaginous polysaccharides such as *Aloe vera*, marshmallow root *Althaea officinalis,* and slippery elm *Ulmus fulva,* and also many seaweeds are often used to improve mucosal health.

These herbs are easiest taken as powders in tablespoonful doses, and can be mixed with stewed apples (peel and all), which contain large amounts of pectin, also a good gut healer.

Marigold *Calendula officinalis* and plantain *Plantago* spp. are both inflam-

Inflammation

mation-mediating herbs excellent at wound healing. A strong decoction of the dried or fresh herbs can be made by simmering them for 20–30 minutes. Ideally this would be drunk on an empty stomach after at least a 12-hour fast. Make the decoction the night before and drink it the next morning. A dose of a handful of the dried herb in about 250ml of water daily would be fine.

Improving digestive function requires the involvement of bitter herbs as well as aromatic digestive herbs.

These should be chosen to suit the person, as ever, with distinctions being made between warming and cooling bitters (see liver herbs above).

Most culinary herbs and spices such as black pepper, mustard, ginger, coriander and cumin will help digestion, and can be taken before eating, with food or afterwards if needed.

If these are not enough, then bitter herbs can be used, ideally before a meal but also useful afterwards. I have a formula for a **digestive bitters tonic**, which has been the most popular formula I have ever made, with hundreds of people finding it useful. This is a mix of bitter herbs and aromatic herbs, which together really help digestion:

- three parts artichoke *Cynara scolymus*
- two parts *Angelica archangelica*
- two parts blessed thistle *Carbenia benedicta*
- one part fennel seed *Foeniculum vulgare*
- one part gentian *Gentiana lutea*
- one part bitter orange peel *Citrus aurantium fr.*
- one part ginger *Zingiber officinale*
- one part centaury *Centaurium erythraea*

Take anything from 20 drops to a teaspoonful of tincture in a little water as needed.

This works best as a tincture as it becomes quite unpleasant if a cup of the tea is drunk. As a tincture it is pleasant to take, if a little bitter to those who are not used to bitter tastes. Everyone gets used to it after a few days.

Further information about all herbs can be found in chapter 9, the materia medica.

The health of the microbiome The human body is an ecosystem, part of which includes a vast number of different microbial organisms that play a vital role in the proper function of our bodies. The role of the gut microbiome is well recognised in the inflammatory process, and the inflammatory process has been shown to have deleterious effects on the microbiome.[21]

It has also been well recognised that pre-industrial peoples have a similar microbiome to each other wherever they live in the world, while those living in industrialised areas have a very different, less healthy microbiome. This is a result of the presence of antibiotics, a diet of processed food, and a much more sanitised environment.

However, there is no such thing as a 'normal' microbiome. This is always individual, so testing to determine a microbiome to see if it is 'healthy' is not that useful. A microbiome will contain not only bacteria, but also viruses, fungi and parasites, and its make-up will be affected by everything from conception onwards. It is considered that the most influence comes from the first one thousand days of life, including time in utero. However, the microbiome can be improved and repaired at all stages of life.

One hundred years ago the killer diseases worldwide were pneumonia, tuberculosis and infectious gut diseases. Nowadays these have been supplanted in the richer, western world by the killer inflammatory diseases – cardiovascular disease, cancer and diabetes. So as a population we have learned how to manage bacteria but in the process overmanaged them so that we killed all microorganisms, beneficial and pathogenic, without the understanding that we actually needed the beneficial ones.

For example, a study has shown that the presence of a bacterium *Blautia obeum* in the gut can protect against cholera by a number of different mechanisms, including its interaction with bile salts. The study found that *B. obeum* was prevalent in the microbiome of people studied in Bangladesh, and that those from Bangladesh had a **very much more diverse microbiome than a similar number of people from the USA.**[22]

The functions of these beneficial microbiota are numerous, and very important to our health. Our understanding of the functions and health of the microbiota have only really developed in recent years, and more and more connections have been drawn between this new industrial microbiota and chronic inflammatory diseases. We still don't know the full story yet but it is developing.[23]

There is evidence that dysbiosis weakens the immune defences, 'thereby predisposing to more severe SARS-CoV-2 infection and contributing to "long COVID"'.[24]

The factor with the most effect on the microbiome is diet, and we need a good variety of foods to feed a large variety of microorganisms. The average modern western diet contains a very small variety of different plant foods, in some cases less than ten, whereas the diet of older generations may well have contained at least one hundred different plant foods.
It is now understood that if we eat at least thirty different plant foods in a week we will have a much healthier microbiome than if we only ate ten different ones. It's actually not that difficult to eat such a variety as plant foods include all grains, nuts, seeds, fruit and vegetables.

One important change in diet from the less developed to the developed world was the reduction of both soluble and insoluble plant fibre-based complex carbohydrates found in plants such as legumes, wholegrains and vegetables. These were replaced by simple carbohydrates, the refined and processed grains and sugar that make up the modern diet, which is much less useful to the microbiome and shown to have altered its structure and function, resulting in dysbiosis (defined as unnatural changes in the composition of the microbiome) and leading to chronic inflammatory disease.

Stress can also have a big impact on the microbiome. This can be physical or mental stress, and can include overworking, sleep deprivation, pollution, local climate change and lack of exercise. Social interaction and physical activity also have an impact on gut and body health.[25]

The microbiome has many important functions, all relevant to the proper function of the immune system, which is the ruling force of inflammation in the body. It can be said to be both a digestive organ and an endocrine organ:

- It resists colonisation by pathogenic organisms.
- It provides information to the immune system to create a healthy balance, that is, homeostasis.
- It can commence inflammation quickly in response to a threat, and shut it down when it has done its job.
- It is essential for the proper function of the gut barrier, which protects the body from anything moving through the gut. So it modulates mucous membranes, which are there to protect cell walls and provide an intact passageway. It modulates the gaps between cells to keep the junctions tight and not allow large molecules to pass into the bloodstream.

- It modulates secretory IgA, the most important antibody found in mucosal secretions and vital in defence of the gut, and often deficient where there are food intolerances.
- It interacts with antimicrobial peptides, which are produced in the intestines to prevent pathogenic microbial growth and infection. These antimicrobial peptides are also essential in shaping the composition of the microbiome.[26]
- It is important for nutrient absorption and creation, particularly vitamin D3, B vitamins and K2, and short chain fatty acids; also electrolyte and water balance.
- It is important for immune tolerance, and avoidance of autoimmune disease.
- It ferments and breaks down indigestible fibres such as inulin and cellulose to short chain fatty acids including butyrate, acetate and propionate, which are required by enterocytes (the cells lining the intestines) for fuel and immune signalling. They also have local and systemic anti-inflammatory properties. Butyrate is also able to signal enterocytes to tighten their junctions.[27]
- A healthy microbiome is linked with healthy brain function. The gut microbiome and the brain have a bidirectional communication.[28]
- A healthy microbiome is linked with healthy skin. Dysbiosis is a cause of inflammatory skin conditions such as psoriasis and eczema.[29]

How to improve microbiome health

There are several ways to improve the microbiome, but it is most important first to improve the health of the gut – improve the terrain. If there is a leaky gut then this needs dealing with first.

The bacteria in the gut microbiome need prebiotics to feed on for their health. The breakdown products of this digestion are short chain fatty acids that are released into the blood circulation and have beneficial effects on the whole body.[30]

They are a particular kind of dietary fibre that is selectively used by the gut microbiota and are vital to the health of the microbiome. Good prebiotic fibre-containing foods include Jerusalem artichokes, apples, bananas, asparagus, leeks, onions, oats, barley and linseeds. Acacia gum and slippery elm *Ulmus fulva* are also excellent prebiotic sources.

Probiotics, the bacteria that can support the microbiome, and can be ingested in capsules or drinks, are useful but are only temporary residents of the gut, and only serve a purpose while they are being taken. In order to encourage the microbiome to flourish the terrain needs to be right, so prebiotics, a healthy diet and a healthy gut wall are most important. Garlic *Allium sativum* is useful as it is a prebiotic, and is antimicrobial towards the pathogenic microorganisms.

Fermented foods and drinks such as sauerkraut, kimchi, kombucha and kefir are most useful here too, and as they are food and drink can be taken daily at much lower cost than probiotic supplements. However, if these are purchased rather than homemade it is important that they are unpasteurised so that the beneficial bacteria are still present. Eating avocados also seems to support healthy gut flora.

Further information about all herbs can be found in chapter 9, the materia medica.

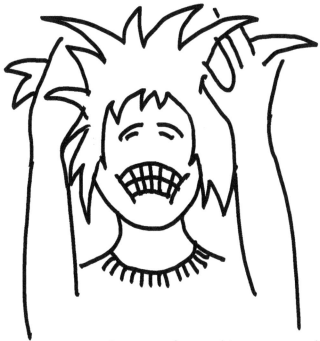

Stress can have a big impact on the microbiome.

The nervous system and inflammation

The nervous system is made up of two main parts, the central nervous system, which includes the brain and spinal cord, and the peripheral nervous system, which includes nerves branching off from the spinal cord and extending to all parts of the body. These nerves carry messages or information in their nerve cells or neurons between the brain and the body and control every action.

There is a strong bi-directional connection between the brain and the gut, via the cranial and the vagus nerve and the peripheral nervous system. So anything that affects the gut will affect the brain and vice versa. When there is an inflammatory state in the gut it will affect the brain, as can be seen in patients with inflammatory bowel diseases such as coeliac disease where there is also a high incidence of brain inflammation visible on an MRI scan.[31]

Or, if the gut is on fire, then the brain will also be on fire.

The action of the vagus nerve is closely linked with inflammatory states in the body.

The vagus nerve, so called because it wanders through the body like a vagabond, originates in the brain, travels down the neck, through the chest to the abdomen, creating an interconnected network between the brain, digestive system, lungs, heart, liver and kidneys. Its main function is to send messages to the brain from the organs so the brain is aware of how they are functioning. The vagus is also able to assess immune function too.

The vagus nerve controls the parasympathetic nervous system, so it is vital in winding down from any sympathetic nervous system activity. The sympathetic nervous system is activated by increased cortisol in the fight-or-flight response created by a stressful situation.

Keeping this balance between parasympathetic and sympathetic is vital for health. Back in the Stone Age it was a matter life or death to have that sympathetic response when we were out hunting, or being hunted, but those who don't deal well with stress and anxiety find themselves in sympathetic mode more or less constantly and unable to revert to relax mode, that is, with parasympathetic dominance.

The sympathetic response releases hormones such as adrenalin and cortisol, resulting in a raised heart rate, tense muscles (ready to run), sweating,

Inflammation

slowed digestion and a feeling of increased energy arising from gluco-neogenesis (the generation of new glucose by the liver). It also releases the hormone renin from the kidneys, which increases blood pressure and increases metabolism. Understanding the stress response is simple if we consider the domestic cat – they are masters of relaxation (parasympa-thetic dominance), but when necessary they can spring into fast action to hunt, or to run from a dog (sympathetic dominance) and then straight back to sleep again afterwards as though nothing had happened.

The sympathetic response releases hormones such as adrenalin and cortisol, resulting in a raised heart rate

Generally the parasympathetic response is anti-inflammatory and the sympathetic response, especially if out of control, is pro-inflammatory. So chronic stress is a major cause of inflammation.

Stress results in the release of inflammatory cytokines through the effect on sympathetic and parasympathetic nervous system pathways. These cytokines have been found to interact with neurotransmitter metabo-lism and neuroendocrine function. Poor sleep results in lowered vagal tone and increased inflammation, and inflammation results in poor sleep. Pro-inflammatory cytokines IL-6 and TNF alpha daytime secretion is increased in insomniacs, which causes more inflammation and contributes to the chronic inflammatory diseases so common today – type 2 diabetes, cancer, osteoarthritis and cardiovascular disease.

How to improve nervous system health

Improving vagal tone will help the body to relax better after any stress. There are several methods of doing this, and the result will reduce inflammation. These techniques need doing long-term and daily for several weeks to get results:

- Cold exposure will activate the vagus nerve, and regular cold exposure can lower the sympathetic response and increase parasympathetic activity via the vagus nerve. This means cold showers, or at least cold face wash.
- Deep and slow breathing activates the vagus nerve, reduces anxiety and increases parasympathetic response. Aim at six breaths a minute as diaphragmatic breathing with expansion of the stomach.
- Singing, humming, chanting and gargling – activates the throat muscles and stimulates the vagus nerve.
- Probiotics – healthy gut bacteria improve brain function by affecting the vagus nerve.

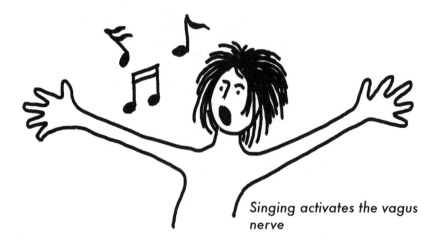

Singing activates the vagus nerve

Inflammation

- Meditation can increase vagal tone.

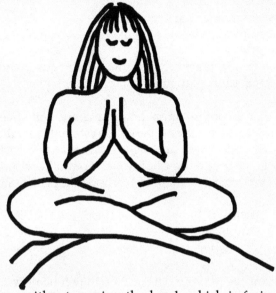

- Eye exercises – without moving the head, which is facing forward, look to the right for one minute, then centre, then left for one minute, breathing slowly as you do it. This can be done sitting or lying down.[32]

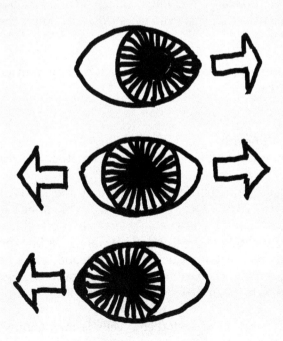

- Omega 3 fatty acids increase vagal tone and vagal activity. For example, oily fish, flaxseed oil, walnuts.
- Exercise stimulates the vagus nerve.
- Massage can stimulate the vagus nerve, as can reflexology and Bowen technique.
- Socialising and laughing stimulate the vagus – and stimulating the vagus often causes laughter.

Anything that causes inflammation in the gut will affect the brain, so in order to protect the brain and nervous system it is vital to follow an anti-inflammatory diet. There are suggestions that non-coeliac gluten sensitivity may be of prime importance here, but all pro-inflammatory foods should be avoided.[33] See chapter 4 for more information.

Plastics, in particular the plasticisers bisphenol A BPA, and bisphenol S BPS, are also implicated in causing inflammatory damage to nerve cells, so avoiding all plastic wraps and bottles is a good move.[34]

Herbs to improve nervous system health will be nervine tonics, nervine relaxants and adaptogens. Many of these double up as inflammation-mediating herbs; notable herbs which do this are chamomile *Matricaria recutita*, lemon balm *Melissa officinalis*, linden flower *Tilia europaeus*, St John's wort *Hypericum perforatum*, skullcap *Scutellaria lateriflora*, ashwagandha *Withania somnifera*, rose root *Rhodiola rosea* and schisandra *Schisandra chinensis*.

Further information about all herbs can be found in chapter 9, the materia medica.

Endothelial cell health
This is another important factor in the inflammatory process.

Endothelial cells form the lining in all blood and lymph vessels in the body. They are there to act as a barrier between blood and lymph and the rest of the body tissues, but also to be selectively permeable to some chemicals to move into body tissues, and permeable to carbon dioxide to move into the bloodstream from tissues. This permeability is a very important function that, among many other things, maintains the blood-brain barrier, which protects the brain from toxic chemicals.

Another main function of endothelial cells is maintaining the elasticity of blood vessels to allow them to constrict and dilate – the processes of

Inflammation

vasoconstriction and vasodilation – in order to control blood flow and blood pressure. Endothelial cells synthesise nitric oxide (NO), which acts as a vasodilator, and also catecholamines, which act as vasoconstrictors. Reduced production and/or bioavailability of NO is considered the central mechanism responsible for endothelial dysfunction.[35] NO also acts as an anticoagulant to prevent anything sticking to the endothelial cell wall.

The endothelium also has a role to play in wound healing by controlling platelet aggregation and as a clotting factor to prevent further bleeding, but is also involved in fibrinolysis, which dissolves clots and prevents thrombosis.

If there is a chronic inflammatory process then damage to the endothelium will result in a loss of elasticity, which results in poor vasodilation and leads to hypertension; also it results in increased incidences of coagulation as it tries to heal itself. This process develops into thrombosis, heart and kidney disease, neurological disease and pulmonary disease. Insulin resistance and diabetes are inflammatory and will also damage the endothelium, hence the link between diabetes and cardiovascular disease.

Endothelial cells lose function with age, diabetes, hypertension, smoking and inactivity. A recent study, looking at mRNA COVID vaccines, concluded that the mRNA vaccines dramatically increase inflammation on the endothelium and T cell infiltration of cardiac muscle, and may account for the observations of increased thrombosis, cardiomyopathy and other vascular events following vaccination.[36]

How to improve the health of the endothelium

- Avoid smoking, inactivity, obesity, sugar and refined carbohydrates.
- Eat more plants, especially wholegrains, nuts and seeds, and drink herb teas, green tea, cocoa and dark chocolate, which all increase endothelial nitric oxide, one of the most helpful ways of supporting the endothelium.
- Spices improve endothelial function, including turmeric, ginger, cinnamon and black pepper.
- Foods to improve microcirculation include chocolate, berries, garlic, beetroot and green tea.

Often the heroic methods of modern medicine – the surgery and medications – are required when heart disease becomes severe, but in the earlier stages, or when things are stabilised, there are plenty of herbal interventions that can help. The main mechanisms of action of the most commonly used hypertension medications are calcium channel blockade, beta adrenergic blockade and angiotensin-converting enzyme inhibition. Herbs have been shown to act by all of these mechanisms as well.

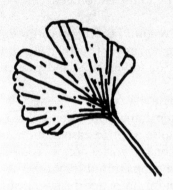 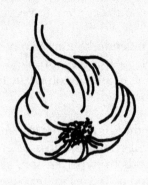

Herbs that will support endothelial function include ginkgo *Ginkgo biloba*, hawthorn *Crataegus oxyacantha*, red sage *Salvia miltiorrhiza*, rose hips *Rosa canina*, reishi *Ganoderma lucidum* and ginger *Zingiber officinale*. Gentian *Gentiana lutea* has been shown to prevent endothelial inflammation.[37]

Further information about all herbs can be found in chapter 9, the materia medica.

Chapter summary:

- chronic inflammation means the whole body needs treating, never just one part of it; the body is a complex network of interdependent parts;
- the immune system explained and how to look after it;
- the digestive system explained and how to look after it – the liver, the gut and the microbiome;
- the nervous system explained and how to look after it;
- endothelial cell function and how to look after it.

4
The causes and risk factors for chronic inflammation

The most important thing is to determine the causative factor of the chronic inflammation. Why is the body having to defend itself – what is attacking it? The name of the resulting disease is less important than the cause of the inflammation and then the inflammation itself. This is where holistic medicine differs from modern allopathic medicine, although there are now signs that modern medicine is learning this.

The 2019 Global Burden of Disease study determined that, after hypertension, the biggest risk factor for attributable deaths for women worldwide was dietary, accounting for 5.25 million deaths annually, which was 20.3% of all female deaths in 2019; the fifth biggest risk factor was high body mass index (BMI).

And for men dietary factors came in third place after smoking and hypertension, causing 4.47 million deaths or 14.6% of all deaths. Malnutrition was a separate risk factor to dietary risks so that total excluded deaths from malnutrition.

The study also looked at disability adjusted life years (DALYs) to see which factors were causing measurable disability problems. It found that, while malnutrition of mothers and children were the highest risk, high BMI, high blood pressure, high blood sugar and dietary risks were the next highest separate risks for both sexes; if these had been considered together as a single risk they would have been by far the greatest risk for both deaths and DALYs. While the metabolic risks were found more in higher-income countries, dietary risks were found at roughly the same level in all socio-demographic index groups (SDI), which was the measurement chosen to assess social and economic development.

The biggest difference between the first global burden of disease study in 1990 and that of 2019 was the number of deaths and DALYs attributable to metabolic disease, namely high BMI, high blood sugar, high blood pressure and dietary risk factors.[1]

The 2017 Global Burden of Disease study looked at the disease-specific burden of each of fifteen food and nutrient groups on non-communicable disease. Their conclusions were that these deaths attributable to diet were too high in sodium and had insufficient whole grains, fruit, vegetables, nuts and seeds and omega 3 fatty acids, and that these were the biggest risk factors both for deaths and DALYs across all SDI groups.[2]

An analysis of the 2017 Global Burden of Disease study in regard to high body mass index found that high BMI caused 2.4 million deaths and 70.7 million DALYs in women, and 2.3 million deaths and 77 million DALYs in men in 2017. These figures had more than doubled between 1990 and 2017, with figures for most high SDI countries decreasing in that time (apart from the USA) and most mid-range SDI countries increasing rapidly in that time. The leading cause of DALYs was cardiovascular disease, followed by diabetes and cancer, together accounting for 89% of all high BMI-related DALYs.

The study concluded that 'the burden of disease imposed by high BMI is particularly dramatic'.[3]

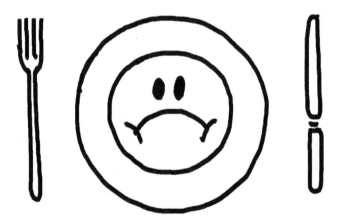

Poor diet

So the number 1 cause of chronic inflammation causing death and disability in the world is poor diet. This is most often combined with one or more of the following factors:

- age
- low sex hormones
- obesity
- poor lifestyle and stress, mental or physical
- poor sleep
- smoking
- inactivity
- dysbiosis
- periodontitis
- poor digestive function
- toxicity, for example heavy metals, agrochemicals, air or water pollution, drugs
- poor elimination of toxins
- unresolved infection

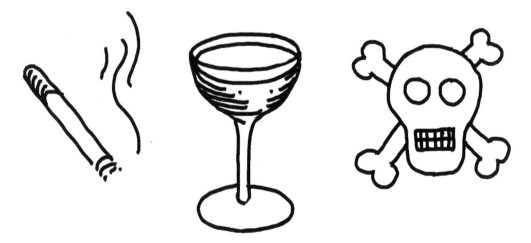

Poor diet – which foods are the problem? The Global Burden of Disease study 2017 found that foods missing from the diet were the most important risk factors – wholegrains, fruit, vegetables, nuts and seeds, and omega 3 fatty acids; but the risk factors they also considered were those that were too high in the diet, including processed and red meat, salt, sugar, and trans fatty acids.

Those missing foods will be considered in more detail in chapter 6, on using diet to reduce inflammation.

There are some foods that cause inflammation in everyone. That doesn't mean they can't be eaten by anyone, it just means that if someone has chronic inflammation these foods should at least be reduced to a minimum, and ideally removed for a month or two to see the effect on the individual. There is more information on each of the following in chapter 6. The inflammatory foods include:

- wheat and gluten grains.
- animal milk products, i.e. dairy.
- alcohol.
- pork and processed meat.
- non grass-fed red meat. This refers mostly to grain-fed beef, which has been shown to produce a greater inflammatory response in comparison to grass-fed beef. Most lamb and mutton is grass-fed, as is the best beef.[4,5]
- sugar: excessive intake of sugar and fructose (especially in the form of high fructose corn syrup) is very inflammatory, and has been linked with inflammation of the endothelial cells lining blood vessels.
- oranges can provoke an inflammatory response in many people, although other citrus fruits are often fine.
- artificial trans fats – these are unsaturated oils that are hydrogenated to create a solid and more stable oil. They are used in processed foods to improve shelf life and are present in many margarines. They are very pro-inflammatory and reduce high-density lipoprotein (HDL) cholesterol, the protective portion of cholesterol that helps to remove the 'bad' LDL cholesterol from the bloodstream. Higher levels of HDL are associated with a lower risk of heart disease.
- some vegetable oils, especially those high in omega 6 oils – e.g. soya bean oil. If a diet is already high in omega 6 fatty acids then adding more will be pro-inflammatory, although a certain amount of omega 6 fatty acids are needed, especially for eye health. Chapter 6 has more information about culinary oils.
- overeating refined carbohydrates can increase pro-inflammatory gut bacteria, leading to obesity and gut inflammation. Refined carbs also have a higher glycaemic index – which causes inflammation, high blood sugar and insulin resistance and eventually diabetes.
- diets high in sugar, refined grains and trans fats are very much associated with chronic inflammatory disease, and particularly with diabetes and metabolic syndrome.

Inflammation

Hayfever case study

A 27-year-old man had severe hayfever, which actually lasted nearly all year. It affected his eyes, nose and throat, and also his lungs. He had been diagnosed with asthma aged 16 months and had been on steroid inhalers ever since. He also had to use strong anti-inflammatory steroidal nasal sprays, antihistamine medication and was on antidepressants too.

He rarely went outside because he was so severely affected by his hayfever, spending most of his time in his room at his parent's house, and he slept during the day as he had trouble sleeping at night. He found it difficult to go to sleep, and when he did sleep he had lots of vivid dreams and nightmares.

His digestion wasn't great and he often had stomach pains.

Very often those with asthma and/or hayfever are intolerant to animal milk protein, and he was no exception. He needed to stop taking any animal milk products containing protein such as cheese, milk and cream. He also needed to start eating vegetables as these didn't feature in his diet at all!

Over the next few months we experimented with several herbs to try and help him wean off some of his medication, and to try and get him a more normal way of life so he could actually venture out of his bedroom and start living. Eventually the best herbal prescription for him was found to be ginger *Zingiber officinale*, black pepper *Piper nigrum* and aniseed *Pimpinella anisum* taken as powders in capsules, together with an antihistaminic formula of Baikal skullcap *Scutellaria baicalensis*, reishi mushroom *Ganoderma lucidum* and plantain *Plantago major* also as powders in a capsule.

He did very well on these herbs, and slept much more normally as long as he stayed off the animal milk products – when he did lapse, as he sometimes did, his asthma symptoms came straight back again.

And then there are the foods that people are intolerant to, which are even more inflammatory in those individuals. It is not always necessary to have digestive symptoms with a food intolerance, and symptoms could include sleep disturbance, skin rashes, bladder irritation, mood swings or even general body heat. The foods and food groups to which someone is intolerant could include:

- animal milk products, i.e. dairy
- wheat and/or gluten grains
- nightshade family foods, i.e. tomatoes, potatoes, peppers and aubergines
- soya-based foods
- high salicylate foods
- high oxalate foods
- high histamine foods
- high lectin foods.

See the box on pages 57–58 for food intolerance testing methods to determine which food is causing inflammation. In my experience, virtually everyone who has a chronic inflammatory condition has a food intolerance to some extent or another. Further information about all the above intolerances can be found in chapter 6.

Food intolerance case study 1

A 58-year-old woman presented with eczema, which had gradually become worse over the previous six months. She had a history of a severe gastro-intestinal infection two years previously and had found that many foods now gave her diarrhoea and stomach ache. She also had hayfever in the summer, which had worsened over the last four years. As a child she had a history of ear infections.

Muscle testing showed intolerance to dairy and high-salicylate foods so she was started on a low-inflammatory diet without dairy and high-salicylate foods.

As it was hayfever season it was suggested that she pick fresh nettle leaf *Urtica dioica* and plantain *Plantago major* to make a herb tea that would reduce her hayfever symptoms. Her skin was not too bad so she decided to try diet alone to see if her skin would improve.

Within three weeks her skin and hayfever were completely better.
Continues on next page

Inflammation

Three years later she came back to see me with osteoarthritis in her thumb joints and hayfever again. As her diet had slipped she was reminded of the need to be dairy- and high salicylate-free and she had a herbal ointment containing comfrey leaf *Symphytum officinale*, arnica *Arnica montana*, calendula *Calendula officinalis* and essential oils of lavender and helichrysum. Within three weeks her thumbs were no longer sore and hayfever was under control again.

Five years later again she returned after being told she had high cholesterol levels and would need to do something about it otherwise she would have to be put on statin medication. It turned out that she had experienced high levels of stress for a couple of years, and although she was sticking to her dairy-free diet, she was now drinking a lot of wine every day. Wine, as it is derived from grapes, is very high in salicylates, so as well as being pro-inflammatory owing to the alcohol content, it was doubly inflammatory to her because of the salicylate content.

So she was reminded about the best diet for her as reducing inflammation is the best approach to result in a lowering of cholesterol. Unfortunately there was no further follow-up, so we'll never know if the new diet made the difference or whether she decided to go on to statin medication.

For more information about diet work and herbs, including a glossary, please see chapters 6 on diet and 9, the materia medica.

Food intolerance case study 2
A 40-year-old man presented with a longstanding cough that had been going on for 15 years and had been investigated and treated by medics to no avail. This was a dry spasmodic cough without phlegm.

No allergies had been found, and he had even tried moving house at one point to see if that was his problem.

He had very few other health problems apart from fatigue, being constantly warm and craving sweet foods. He snacked a great deal on sweet snacks.

Continues on next page

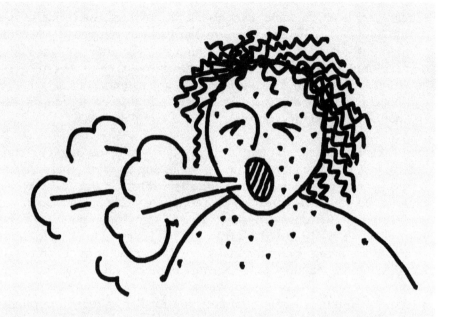

Muscle testing indicated dairy intolerance so he was started on a low-inflammation dairy-free diet and given a herbal tincture containing:

- Elecampane *Inula helenium*, an antitussive bronchodilator and lung tonic
- Self heal *Prunella vulgaris*, a cooling inflammation-mediating vulnerary often used for throat and mouth problems
- White horehound *Marrubium vulgare*, an antispasmodic expectorant often used for coughing
- Holy basil *Ocimum sanctum*, an inflammation-mediating bronchodilator, vulnerary and adaptogen
- *Lobelia inflata*, an antispasmodic targeting the respiratory tract.

Within three weeks his cough had gone. He stayed on the herbs for about six weeks altogether but then no longer needed them.

For more information about diet work and herbs, including a glossary, please see chapters 6 on diet and 9, the materia medica.

Testing for food intolerances

There are several methods of testing which food is causing the problem.

- The first is to guess at the most likely cause from the symptom pattern or from any known history in the family, and remove it for long enough to observe any changes. This is the elimination method. See below for some of the symptom pictures that can give clues to which foods to try.
- Another method that can be used, and that I personally use in my clinic, with I believe a 99 per cent success rate, is to muscle-test. All the case studies mentioned here were tested by this method. This is a test that has to be seen and used to be believed, and there is no scientific backing for it, but it does work. It is a method of asking the body what it likes and doesn't like, and results are very clear. To do this you may need to find someone who uses applied kinesiology (muscle testing) as a therapy, but anyone can do it with some practice. The food that comes up as a problem can then be removed from the diet with more certainty than the elimination method, and if digestive symptoms improve then all is good. It just makes everything quicker and easier.
- Anyone tested in my clinic will have had a detailed medical history taken, together with clinical observations. They will then be muscle-tested for all major food groups and will then be given a specific diet programme. They are asked to return in around three weeks so they can be followed up, but can get in touch in the meantime if necessary. I have found this four-pronged approach – observation, medical history, muscle testing and then removal of foods found – to be amazingly accurate.
- A further method that can be used is a pulse test – when a substance is ingested that upsets the body very often there is a rise in pulse. So take a pulse rate before and after ingestion of the test substance.
- It is also sometimes possible to put a small amount of the substance on the skin, make sure it stays there (with a small bandage, for example) and observe for any reddening of the skin over some hours. This last method works if someone has a strong intolerance or allergy, but I don't think it is so sensitive otherwise.
- Commercial testing of blood for antibodies to specific foods. The people selling these tests admit that they get lots of false positives, and people end up with a list of twenty or thirty different foods that they have to cut out, when in reality it may only be one food group.

Continues on next page

There have been recent advances in testing that actually look to see which foods create inflammation as well as which antibodies to foods are present, but this is relatively expensive and, in my experience of several thousand patients, any of the above testing is just as good and far cheaper.

There are certain patterns of symptoms that can show which food is worth excluding first if you are trying the elimination method of testing.

If someone has a lot of mucus and phlegm, with catarrh, sinus congestion, continual throat clearing and a history of tonsillitis and/or ear infections, sometimes with seasonal hayfever, then dairy exclusion is the first thing to try. This is also the case with hormonal imbalance or disease, for men and women.

If there is a pattern of repeated urinary tract infections, and maybe bladder irritation or a history of bedwetting, then dairy is also likely, but salicylate sensitivity has to be considered too.

A history of headaches with constipation and sometimes joint stiffness and pain, and skin rashes can suggest nightshade family sensitivity.

Wheat and gluten sensitivity can show symptoms of skin rashes, and also digestive problems such as diarrhoea or bloating.

None of these are definitive pictures of a food sensitivity or intolerance, but they can guide you to eliminating a particular food first, which will save time and stress.

Age – inflammaging
Inflammaging is the term that describes the process of increasing inflammation with increasing age. Epidemiological studies have found that inflammaging is a risk factor for cardiovascular disease, cancer, chronic kidney disease, dementia and depression as well as disability and early death.[6]

Studies have found several stimuli for inflammaging, including persistent viral infections such as cytomegalovirus or coronavirus (COVID-19), or bacterial infection such as seen in periodontitis. Also the aging immune system can become less efficient at clearing cell debris or oxidised proteins. The gut microbiota is crucially important in this process because it

Inflammaging is the term that describes the process of increasing inflammation with increasing age

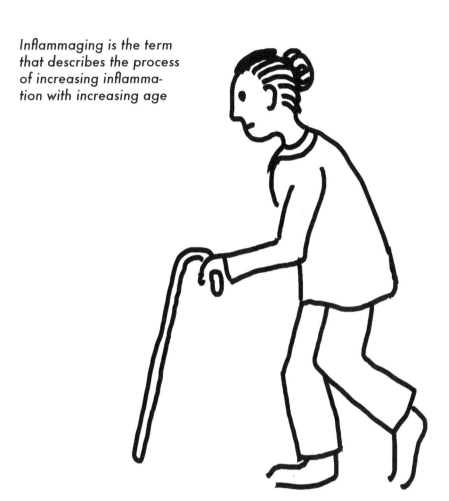

interfaces with diet, metabolism and the immune response, and because it changes with age.[7]

Studies have shown that there are two factors in particular that can ameliorate inflammaging. One is calorie restriction (which can be overall restriction or intermittent fasting); and the other is when body core temperature is lowered, for example, in hibernation.[8] Intermittent fasting is discussed in chapter 6.

Sex hormones, in particular oestrogen and testosterone, can inhibit production of some pro-inflammatory markers, reducing the incidence of inflammatory disease. With increasing age, these sex hormones decrease, so as part of inflammaging low levels of oestrogen and testosterone result in inflammation.

The causes and risk factors for chronic inflammation   59

Obesity and metabolic disease

Many studies have shown the link between increased body fat and the amount of secreted pro-inflammatory cytokines and other inflammatory mediators.

Obesity itself can cause inflammation – fat tissue can be termed an endocrine organ that secretes inflammatory cytokines and other inflammatory chemicals such as adipokines. Central or abdominal obesity seems to be most associated with inflammation, and the greater the size of the fatty tissue the greater the inflammation. Weight loss, exercise and calorie restriction are associated with reduction in pro-inflammatory markers and improvement in cardiovascular risk.[10,11]

Metaflammation is defined as low-grade, chronic inflammation orchestrated by metabolic cells in response to excess nutrients and energy. Metabolic diseases include insulin resistance, diabetes, cardiovascular diseases

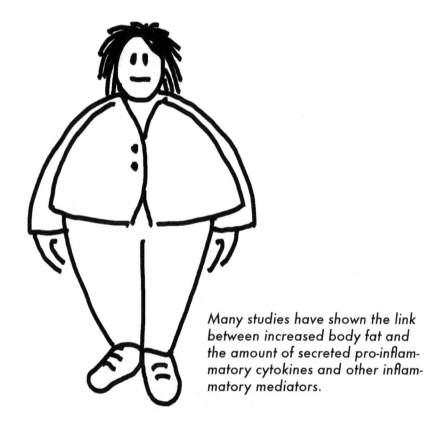

Many studies have shown the link between increased body fat and the amount of secreted pro-inflammatory cytokines and other inflammatory mediators.

Inflammation

and obesity, which are all caused by and cause chronic inflammation. When there is nutrient overload, especially when food is too high in pro-inflammatory fatty acids, the innate immune system is overstimulated. Immune cells become unable to function properly and this results in metabolic disorders.[12]

The hormone ghrelin has an important role in both obesity and metabolic disorders. Ghrelin has long been known as the hormone produced by the body in response to hunger. It signals the need to eat, and is reduced when food has been eaten. However, it has been found that ghrelin also has a role in insulin management and chronic inflammation,[13] as well as in reducing sympathetic nervous system activity.[14]

Stress, physical and mental
Stress is associated with increased chronic inflammation. This highlights the interconnections between emotions, the nervous system and the immune system, termed psychoneuroendocrinology.

Stress is often linked with poor sleep patterns, which are another cause of chronic inflammation. This becomes a vicious circle with the increased inflammation resulting in poor sleep. Pro-inflammatory cytokines IL-6 and TNF alpha daytime secretion is increased in insomniacs. The cycle needs to be broken by treating inflammation and cytokine production during the day and sedating at night.

Stress results in release of inflammatory cytokines through the effect on sympathetic and parasympathetic nervous system pathways. These cytokines have been found to interact with neurotransmitter metabolism and neuroendocrine function.[15]

It has also been shown that stress can disrupt the blood–brain barrier, allowing inflammatory molecules, infective agents and toxins to access the brain, causing damage.[16]

Lack of exercise
Human studies have shown that regular exercise, even as little as 20 minutes a day, reduces inflammation even if there is no weight loss.

Regular exercise has a protective role against chronic metabolic and cardiovascular disease, due, to one extent or another, to its anti-inflammatory effects. These include increased catecholamine levels, which inhibit LPS stimulated inflammation markers; tumour necrosis factor (TNF); inhibition of adipose tissue infiltration by monocytes and macrophages;

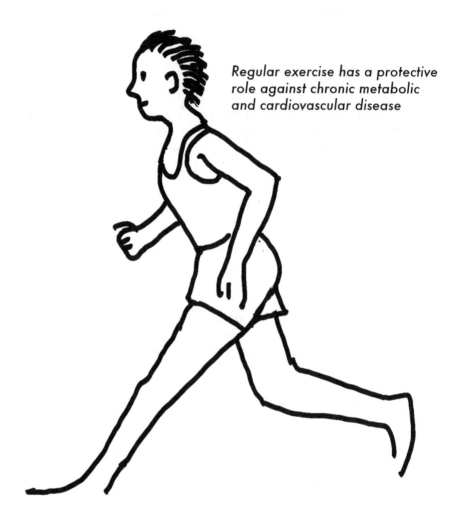

Regular exercise has a protective role against chronic metabolic and cardiovascular disease

reduced expression of Toll-like receptors on monocytes and macrophages; and an increase in the circulating numbers of T regulatory cells.[17]

Dysbiosis
Dysbiosis is the term for unnatural changes in the composition of the microbiome, which might be caused by antibiotic medication, poor diet or intestinal infection of some kind. Dysbiosis affects the immune system and creates inflammation. A healthy microbiota is actually anti-inflammatory. This has been explored in more detail in chapter 3.

Inflammation

Case study

A 32-year-old woman presented with upper respiratory tract inflammation, coughing, wheezing and hayfever. She had a long history of chronic fatigue, going back 24 years, which had started after the flu. She had been bedridden for two years as a child, and had been ill until she was around 18 years old. The previous year she had been put on antibiotics for six months for acne, which followed her menstrual cycle. The acne had improved but was still present.

Muscle testing showed she was intolerant to dairy products and soya, so she was asked to exclude these from her diet and start on an anti-inflammatory diet.

She was started on probiotics to attempt the repair of her gut microbiome. This was the likely cause of her new symptoms. Vitamins D3 and C and magnesium were also given.

Herbs were chosen to help with acne and as inflammation mediators for her upper respiratory tract, although the best treatment for the latter was the combination of probiotics and diet.

Her herbal formula was:

- Figwort *Scrophularia nodosa*, an alterative acting on the lymph and liver
- Yellow dock *Rumex officinalis*, an alterative acting on the lymph and liver
- Oregon grape *Mahonia aquifolium*, an alterative acting on the lymph, liver and skin
- Pleurisy root *Asclepias tuberosa*, an inflammation-mediating antispasmodic herb acting on the lungs
- Liquorice root *Glycyrrhiza glabra*, an inflammation-mediating demulcent, bronchodilator and adaptogen, which also improves the flavour of herbal tinctures.

She also had a herb tea containing:

- Plantain *Plantago major*, a demulcent and decongesting bronchodilator useful in allergies
- Eyebright *Euphrasia officinalis*, an inflammation-mediating decongestant and demulcent

Continues on next page

- Eucalyptus *Eucalyptus globulus*, a decongestant bronchodilator
- Goldenrod *Solidago virgaurea*, an inflammation-mediating decongestant and vulnerary.

Her cough and upper respiratory symptoms improved very quickly with her diet changes, but over the next few years she often needed support for her chronic fatigue. The acne resolved within about six months and with her new diet didn't cause any more problems. However, any stress, physical or mental, resulted in coughing and very low energy levels. Over the years the herbs were changed often to fit her current symptoms, but regular herbs that helped her were:

- Lobelia *Lobelia inflata*, an antispasmodic specific for the upper respiratory tract for coughing
- Ashwagandha *Withania somnifera*, an inflammation-mediating adaptogen
- Astragalus *Astragalus membranaceus*, an inflammation-mediating adaptogen
- Angelica *Angelica archangelica*, an inflammation-mediating tonic herb
- Reishi mushroom *Ganoderma lucidum*, an adaptogen very useful in reducing histamine allergic reactions.

For more information about diet work and herbs, including a glossary, please see chapters 6 on diet and 9, the materia medica.

Periodontal disease

This is a chronic inflammatory disease affecting the periodontium, which includes the gums, ligaments and bone holding the teeth. While its incidence in the UK has decreased over the last few decades, most people have gingivitis, and advanced periodontitis affects 5–15 per cent of the population. Many more have less advanced periodontitis.[18]

The mouth also has a microbiome, consisting of up to 700 different varieties of bacteria, which all need to be in balance just as the gut microbiome. If it tips out of balance then dysbiosis occurs and a low-grade chronic inflammatory state follows, initially in the mouth and then the digestive system and into the whole body. There are many possible causes of oral dysbiosis, which include:

- poor diet
- poor oral hygiene, causing a build-up of plaque, which prevents oxy-

Inflammation

gen from getting to lower layers and results in proliferation of pathogenic anaerobic bacteria
- antibiotics
- mouthwashes
- anything that causes a dry mouth (xerostomia) such as medication or disease, particularly autoimmune disease
- smoking[19]

Those with periodontitis have increased inflammatory markers, and there is a bidirectional link with other forms of chronic inflammation, so that an increase in one creates an increase in the other.[20]

The pro-inflammatory markers will spread throughout the body causing vascular lesions and inflammation.[21] For those with periodontitis there is a:

- 25% increased risk of cardiovascular disease and a 20% increased risk of hypertension[22]
- x 3 risk of diabetes[23]
- x 3 risk of obesity[24]
- 70% increased risk of Alzheimer's disease[25]

Poor digestive function
Poor digestive function, including poor liver function, results in chronic inflammation. The liver is also very involved with the metabolism of sex hormones such as testosterone and oestrogen, and when these are low there is a higher risk of chronic inflammatory disease. The tight junctions between cells lining the gut wall can become loose, creating leaky gut and allowing through large molecules that cause more damage. This has been explored in more detail in chapter 3.

Unresolved low grade viral, bacterial, fungal or parasitic infection
While such unresolved infection has been mentioned as a contributing cause to inflammaging, this can have an impact on the body at any age. It is particularly commonly seen in many cases of chronic fatigue where there is often an underlying low-grade infection that the body cannot fight; it is also seen in human immunodeficiency virus (HIV) infection and other similar infections.

It seems to be involved in post-COVID-19 infections too where there is a prolonged lack of recovery. If the immune system was strong it would have resolved the infection.

Often people with this feel as though they are getting a cold, they might have a throat tickle, or feel a bit achey, but it never really develops. When they finally do have a 'proper' cold with copious sneezing, runny nose and temperature, then they are truly recovering as their immune system is finally able to mount a real response.

Toxicity

Toxicity can arise from tobacco use, agrochemical use, in the workplace or home chemicals. Toxic chemicals can suppress or overload the immune system and cause or increase inflammation. If there is already inflammation present then susceptibility will increase.

It is known that exposure to certain chemicals, including benzene, halocarbons, ketones and nitrosamines, can result in inflammatory diseases such as hepatitis, nephritis, scleroderma and lupus. This is due to production of reactive oxygen species (ROS) by the chemical, or by immune reaction. This can develop into chronic inflammatory diseases such as Alzheimer's disease and cancer.[26]

Neurotoxic metals such as mercury from amalgam, cadmium or lead are associated with excessive levels of ROS together with increased inflammation markers. This is particularly relevant to age-related neurodegenerative disease.[27]

Mercury from amalgam fillings can continuously corrode, releasing mercury into the body. The body can remove it, but only slowly and only if it is functioning well and efficiently. So if there is already a chronic inflammatory disease then detoxification will be impaired. If mercury does build up in the body it will create a constant low-grade inflammation, by dysregulation of cytokine signalling pathways, particularly affecting the nervous system.[28]

Mercury toxicity has been implicated in chronic inflammatory diseases such as cardiovascular disease, allergies, depression and autoimmune diseases such as lupus, graves, Hashimotos and rheumatoid arthritis. It also appears that mercury can disrupt the microbiome and the gut lining, creating dysbiosis and further inflammation.[29]

Mercury toxicity affects mitochondrial function and increases oxidative stress, and results, among other problems, in endothelial dysfunction, dyslipidaemia and immune dysfunction. The consequences of mercury toxicity include hypertension, atherosclerosis, stroke and kidney disease.[30]

Inflammation

Poor elimination

If the body is healthy and functioning as it should do, none of these causes of toxicity would be a problem as an efficient eliminatory system would get rid of them. In small amounts they wouldn't really be noticed, but when there is a build-up over months or years, owing to poor elimination then they cause chronic inflammatory disease.

There are several systems in the body that should do this process.

First, the skin is the largest organ in the body, which forms a protective barrier between our insides and the outside world. It also has the ability to excrete via the sweat and sebaceous glands and is an important organ of elimination. As an eliminative organ it is able to metabolise and eliminate many water-soluble xenobiotic substances such as heavy metals, organic pollutants and medications. It can also eliminate excess lipids via sebaceous glands, and it has a reactive oxygen species (ROS) scavenging system, contributing to the body's antioxidant capacity.

It has been estimated that there are between three and four million sweat glands distributed over the skin surface, which can excrete several litres

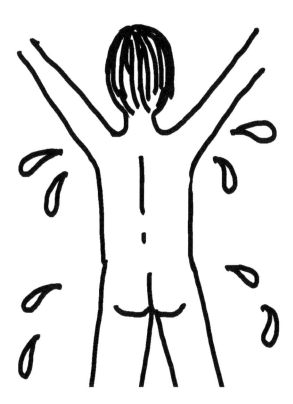

The causes and risk factors for chronic inflammation

an hour when needed. Using a sauna to increase sweating can protect against oxidative stress and metabolic disease. There is evidence that reduced skin elimination function is linked with the metabolic syndrome inflammatory disorders because of toxicity that creates inflammation.[31]

Second, the kidneys are also important in excretion of water-soluble toxic elements. They filter the blood and excrete urea and excess fluids from the body, making sure that the fluid balance in the body is correct. Urea is water-soluble high-nitrogen waste from the liver which, if not removed, would cause serious problems. The kidneys also release hormones that control blood pressure.

Third, the bowels are the organ of elimination that remove all the solid waste left over after the process of digestion and absorption. If the bowels are sluggish there will be toxins present that should have been eliminated such as indoles, phenols and skatoles. If there is constipation or irritation causing diarrhoea the bowel flora will be adversely affected and the bowels will be unable to do their job properly.

Fourth, with regard to elimination, the liver processes and detoxifies hormones, drugs, chemicals and alcohol – basically anything that might be toxic to the body. It does this by filtering the blood to remove large toxins, and by creating bile, which will dissolve the fat-soluble toxins, and lastly by the use of enzymes in two phases involving oxidation and conjugation, it will metabolise toxins into less toxic chemicals. Any nitrogen-containing amino acids are converted to urea, and all these can then be eliminated by the kidneys or bowels.

Fifth, the lungs are another organ of elimination. They eliminate carbon dioxide from the blood that has been brought to the lungs via the heart and circulation. They are able to filter out and eliminate inhaled particles including pathogenic microorganisms using their mucous membranes and cilia, and using macrophages specific to the lungs that are able to recognise foreign bodies.

Sixth, good circulation, both of blood and lymph, is also vital in elimination and detoxification; as are sufficient fluids to allow removal of water-soluble toxins. Lymph is part of the immune system, a clear fluid that carries immune cells to sites of infection, carries nutrients to body cells, and removes waste from them, taking the waste to the blood circulation where it will be disposed of by the other elimination systems of the body.

Alterative herbs are the herbs of choice to improve elimination in the body, and in treating chronic inflammation they are a vital first step in order to be successful. This is not a case of improving elimination by force as the heroic physicians of the past have done with bloodletting, emetics and purgatives. It is important to choose herbs that are right for the individual, which will support the natural elimination systems of the body. As Peter Holmes so beautifully puts it, 'we need to assess and honour the body's own intrinsic ability to bring itself to balance' in choosing eliminative herbs.[32] See box following.

Alterative herbs

Alterative herbs increase elimination of waste products from the body by making the process more effective. We have elimination systems – kidneys, liver, lungs, lymph, bowels and skin – for getting rid of waste products, and any of them can get sluggish and inefficient. Waste products include the normal end products of metabolism in the body as well as toxins that have arrived accidentally. Most alteratives are stimulating, but they are not purely stimulants, they have other functions too.

<u>Alteratives to support the kidneys.</u> These diuretic herbs have an influence upon water excretion via the kidneys and help to drain fluids from the body.

- Burdock *Arctium lappa*
- Celery seed *Apium graveolens*
- Cleavers *Galium aparine*
- Dandelion leaf *Taraxacum officinale*
- Nettle leaf *Urtica dioica*
- Yarrow *Achillea millefolium*

<u>Alteratives to support the liver.</u> Hepatic herbs are primarily bitter tonics, which also stimulate digestion. It is important to choose the right one as some stimulate the liver and some calm it down while improving function. This distinction can be very important – give a person with eczema stimulant liver herbs and they may have a severe flare-up of their skin condition. Use calming liver herbs, and the effects on the liver will be as good, although they may take a little longer, but people shouldn't experience the flare-up. See table in chapter 3.

- Artichoke leaf *Cynara scolymus* (stimulating)
- Burdock *Arctium lappa* (calming)
- Calendula *Calendula officinalis* (stimulating)
- Dandelion root *Taraxacum officinale* (calming)
- Fringe tree *Chionanthus virginicus* (stimulating)

- Goldenseal *Hydrastis canadensis* (stimulating)
- Oregon grape *Mahonia aquifolium* (stimulating)
- St John's wort *Hypericum perforatum* (calming)
- Yarrow *Achillea millefolium* (calming)
- Yellow Dock *Rumex crispus* (stimulating)

Alteratives to support the lymphatic system. These herbs help to drain the lymph and prevent stagnation. Many will also influence immunity, as the immune system is strongly rooted in the lymph.

- Blue flag *Iris versicolor*
- Calendula *Calendula officinalis*
- Cleavers *Galium aparine*
- Echinacea *Echinacea purpurea, E. angustifolia*
- Figwort *Scrophularia nodosa*
- Poke *Phytolacca decandra*
- Red clover *Trifolium pratense*
- Wild indigo *Baptisia tinctoria*

Alteratives to support the gastrointestinal system. Hepatic alteratives are also going to act to improve overall digestion and bowel function as they are all bitter herbs. But there are also the stimulant laxatives. These should only be used short-term, unlike most of the other alteratives listed here.

Stimulant laxatives include

- Cascara sagrada *Rhamnus purshiana*
- Rhubarb root *Rheum* spp.
- Senna *Senna alexandrina*

Alteratives to support the skin. These are herbs that are commonly used for chronic skin conditions such as eczema to improve skin function and elimination. They must be used cautiously with inflammatory skin conditions as they can cause a flare-up if too much pressure is placed on the skin. They should be used alongside alteratives to improve both kidney, bowel and liver function.

- Burdock *Arctium lappa*
- Calendula *Calendula officinalis*
- Cleavers *Galium aparine*
- Dandelion root *Taraxacum officinale*

Inflammation

- Oregon grape *Mahonia aquifolium*
- Red clover *Trifolium pratense*
- Sarsaparilla *Smilax* spp.
- Yellow dock *Rumex crispus*.

Diaphoretic alteratives. These herbs help to promote sweating during fever, but can also be used for detoxification through the skin.

- Boneset *Eupatorium perfoliatum*
- Cayenne *Capsicum annuum*
- Elderflower *Sambucus nigra*
- Garlic *Allium sativum*

Alteratives to support the circulatory system. These are really circulatory stimulants. Some are more specific for detoxification, but in general increasing circulation during alterative therapy is critical to keep everything moving through the system and to the channels of elimination.

- Cayenne *Capsicum annuum*
- Garlic *Allium sativum*
- Ginger *Zingiber officinale*
- Prickly ash *Zanthoxylum americanum*
- Rosemary *Salvia Rosmarinus*
- Sarsaparilla *Smilax* spp.

Alteratives to support the lungs and respiratory system. These herbs are often expectorants and antimicrobials as well.

- Garlic *Allium sativum*
- Echinacea *Echinacea purpurea, E. angustifolia*
- Elderberry and elderflower *Sambucus nigra*
- Elecampane *Inula helenium*
- Mullein *Verbascum thapsus*
- Wild indigo *Baptisia tinctoria*

The contraindication for alteratives is if someone is very dry, although it may be enough to add moistening herbs such as marshmallow *Althaea officialis* or to make sure they get enough fluids. But if people start having any problems with constipation, dry mouth or dry skin then it may be necessary to reduce the dose or have a break from alteratives.

More information about all these herbs can be found in chapter 9, the materia medica.

The causes and risk factors for chronic inflammation

Chapter summary:
It is vital to determine the cause(s) in order to treat the problem, otherwise no real solution will be found. The main cause worldwide of chronic inflammation has been shown to be poor diet. But there will be other factors combined with this:

- diet including food intolerances and testing for them
- age
- low sex hormones
- obesity
- poor lifestyle and stress, mental or physical
- poor sleep
- smoking
- inactivity
- dysbiosis
- periodontitis
- poor digestive function
- toxicity, for example heavy metals, agrochemicals, air or water pollution, drugs
- poor elimination of toxins
- unresolved infection

There is a section on alterative herbs – herbs that improve the eliminatory functions of the body.

5
The results of inflammation – the chronic inflammatory diseases

Chronic inflammation is the underlying reason for all the major non-communicable diseases we see today. It is the result of the many different pathological processes described in the chapters above, which result in tissue stagnation, damage and malfunction.

Chronic inflammation especially involves the digestive system, with its relatively fast cell turnover and its proximity to the damaging elements of digestion. This all leads to low mood, low energy, obesity, lowered immunity and eventually the chronic inflammatory diseases:

* allergies
* arthritis
* autoimmune diseases
* bladder inflammation
* cancer
* cardiovascular disease
* chronic fatigue and fibromyalgia
* diabetes and metabolic diseases
* inflammatory and irritable gut diseases
* inflammatory lung diseases
* inflammatory skin diseases
* neurodegenerative disease
* mental health problems
* osteoporosis
* chronic pain.

There is an epidemic of chronic inflammatory diseases worldwide, with incidences increasing all the time and mostly related to changing lifestyles. Instead of dying suddenly of acute infections we now die more slowly of chronic inflammatory diseases.

There are many factors that interact to lead to chronic inflammatory disease. Our genes determine our individual strengths and weaknesses, but epigenetics determines how our genes express themselves, and the way we live our life will influence this. Variable factors include diet, our personal environment, and the health of our gut microbiome, our digestive system and our immune system. So blaming a chronic disease on family history is not good enough – it is perfectly possible to change gene expression with diet and lifestyle.

Although chronic inflammation progresses silently, it is the cause of most chronic diseases and presents a major threat to the health and longevity of individuals.[1]

The disease states examined in this chapter are only briefly described because everyone's experience of a named disease will be different, leading to different treatments that will almost certainly need to be explored with a therapist. The aim of this chapter is simply to give an overall picture of the links between inflammation and each disease, and to illustrate some of the diseases with case studies.

Allergies
There is a persistent spiral of inflammation, tissue damage and allergy that is now very pervasive and is regularly seen even in children. Most allergic disease reflects the long-term consequences of chronic allergic inflammation.[2]

The health of the gut is very closely linked with allergies and intolerances, with the microbiome and gut wall integrity being paramount. Once food intolerances are dealt with it is surprising just how many other allergies improve. The analogy can be seen as a bucket into which allergens and pro-inflammatory molecules flow, and when there are too many, the bucket will overflow. This overflow becomes the symptoms of the allergies. So if we can reduce the allergens and inflammatory molecules then the body can cope with the load it has.

A very common combination is that of hayfever and animal milk intolerance. Once animal milk is removed from the diet suddenly hayfever symptoms disappear. Similarly many people with asthma find their symptoms disappear, or at least reduce, when they remove animal milk products from their diet.

Multiple allergies case study 1

A 41-year-old woman presented with multiple allergies. Allergy testing by the NHS had found her to suffer from allergies to cats, timothy grass, house dust and dogs. For her the allergies resulted in eczema, rhinitis, hayfever and severe skin itching.

She also had a mild irritable bowel with heartburn and loose bowels. Her energy was low and quite often she felt depressed. Recent blood tests showed slightly abnormal liver function tests, which was her trigger to try and sort herself out by seeing a herbalist.

Her medications were fexofenadine, an antihistamine, and sertraline, an antidepressant.

On muscle testing she was found to be intolerant to dairy products and high-salicylate foods.

As well as diet work she was started on a herbal formula of:

- Milk thistle *Silybum marianum*, a liver-protective herb and inflammation mediator
- Baical skullcap *Scutellaria baicalensis*, an inflammation mediator very useful in reducing histaminic allergic reactions
- Reishi mushroom *Ganoderma lucidum*, an adaptogen very useful in reducing histaminic allergic reactions.

Within four weeks she reported better energy levels, improvements in digestion, skin and rhinitis. Another month later her liver function test was now normal, she was off anti-histamine medication and found she didn't need the herbs any more. Diet alone was keeping her well. She felt strong enough to start withdrawing from the sertraline.

I didn't see her after this but hopefully the outcome was positive. Often people just need help to get over the first difficult stages, then they are strong enough to continue their health journey by themselves.

For more information about diet work and herbs, including a glossary, please see chapters 6 on diet and 9, the materia medica.

Multiple allergies case study 2

A 23-year-old woman presented with repeated bladder infections, which occurred at least once every six weeks and required antibiotics to treat them. She had a history of severe allergies since infancy. She had found that moving to live in sunnier climes had helped her to cope with her allergies better.

Her allergic reactions were to very many things and resulted in asthma, eczema and swelling all over her body and face. She was suffering with Sjogren's syndrome and also had Reynaud's disease and Gilbert's syndromes.

She was always cold, but easily sweaty, and craved cold drinks and ice. She had been using a steroid (beclometasone) inhaler to prevent asthma since she was 18 months old. She had a history of ear infection and had constant vaginal thrush.

She was taking sea buckthorn oil to help the Sjogren's and cranberry to help her bladder infections.

Muscle testing indicated intolerance to dairy, soya, egg, high-salicylate foods and high-histamine foods.

As both sea buckthorn and cranberry are high in salicylates she was advised to stop these.

She was started on a low-inflammation diet, dairy-, egg- and soya-free, low in salicylates and histamines. This was a very restricted diet, but it should be short term for some of the elements. Once the inflammation was reduced and her gastrointestinal tract could start to heal it would be possible to increase the foods she could eat.

She was prescribed a tea for her bladder:

- Marshmallow leaf *Althaea officinalis*, a demulcent inflammation-mediating herb, healing to irritated mucous membranes
- Couch grass root *Agropyron repens*, a demulcent inflammation-mediating herb
- Corn silk *Zea mays*, a demulcent inflammation-mediating herb.

Suggested supplements were L-glutamine to heal the gut, gentle probiotics to replace microbiome (fermented foods are high in histamine so she couldn't have these), vitamin C and D3, magnesium and a multivitamin. Also cider vinegar topically to treat thrush.

Over the next three years she was able to slowly reintroduce eggs, soya, high-histamine and high-salicylate foods and her bladder was very much

Inflammation

improved, without any more infections. She stayed on the bladder tea all this time as she felt it was helpful. Her eyes were much better and her Sjogren's improved a great deal, but she still had occasional flare-ups of allergic reactions, which were not so bad when she lived abroad instead of the UK.

For more information about diet work and herbs, including a glossary, please see chapters 6 on diet and 9, the materia medica.

Arthritis
Osteoarthritis used to be termed non-inflammatory, while rheumatoid and reactive arthritis were termed inflammatory. However, it seems that osteoarthritis is a mixture of degeneration and inflammation in most cases. This fits with the clinical experience of herbalists as osteoarthritis is very treatable with inflammation-mediating herbs and diet. It is not simply a 'wear and tear' disorder of joints.[3]

Rheumatoid arthritis is autoimmune in origin, so determining the underlying cause is very important in order to be able to treat it. See section on autoimmune disease below.

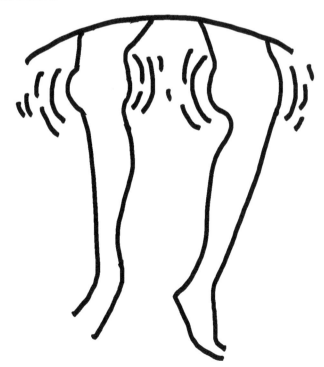

Arthritis case study

A 45-year-old woman presented with inflammation in many joints and connective tissue. She had tendonitis, bursitis and joint pains in shoulders, elbows, hands, feet and knees, giving her limited movement, pain and swelling. She had been diagnosed with arthritis when aged 12.

She also had asthma, eczema, allergic rhinitis, and bladder frequency and urgency with regular cystitis.

She was on lots of inflammation-suppressing medication including beconase, ventolin and phyllocontin for asthma; prednisolone for her joints; cetirizine (an antihistamine) for the allergic rhinitis and dermovate for eczema. She had a history of multi-antibiotic use for chest infections since childhood.

She frequently felt very hot and had a dry mouth and cracked tongue. Both are signs of heat and inflammation with a drying out of fluids.

She was already taking a few supplements, including fish oils, probiotics and a multivitamin.

On muscle testing she was found to be intolerant to dairy products and high-salicylate foods.

As well as diet work she was started on an inflammation-mediating herbal formula of:

- Devil's claw *Harpagophytum procumbens*, primarily for joints, an inflammation-mediating alterative
- Guduchi *Tinospora cordifolia*, primarily for joints, an inflammation-mediating alterative
- Goldenrod *Solidago virgaurea*, for bladder, rhinitis and asthma
- Yarrow *Achillea millefolium*, for general inflammation-mediating, bitter and cooling
- Sweet violet *Viola odorata*, cooling and supports the respiratory tract and skin
- Centaury *Centaurium erythraea*, bitter, cooling and supports the digestive tract.

I had contact with her on and off over the next six years during which she took the same herbs every now and again for a couple of months at a time. She followed her diet and slowly managed to wean herself off all medications, and became very well. This was a well-motivated woman, who really sorted herself out. I met very many people on these kinds of multi-medications who slowly went downhill, adding more and more medications and never managing to gain the upper hand.

For more information about diet work and herbs, including a glossary, please see chapters 6 on diet and 9, the materia medica.

Autoimmune disease

Where the immune system breaks down and starts attacking self tissue cells as being 'foreign', the resulting autoimmune disease include multiple sclerosis (MS), rheumatoid arthritis (RA), coeliac disease and lupus; there is also increasing evidence to show that abnormal inflammatory response is responsible for autoimmune disease.[4]

Development of autoimmune disease requires both a primary lesion and immune dysregulation. The primary lesion could be infection, gut wall damage or some other cause of chronic inflammation. The immune dys-regulation can be any of the causes of inflammation so far discussed such as stress, dysbiosis, obesity, toxicity and so on.

Some peptides in foods are identical to peptides in body tissue. For example, wheat contains some identical peptides to those in collagen. So if there is an immunological reaction to a food, creating antibodies against that food, those antibodies will also attack the body tissue. This is called molecular mimicry.

Cross-reactive peptides have been identified in milk, corn, soya, eggs and some nuts. Molecular mimicry is found between various infective microorganisms and human tissue, the idea being that the microorganism can invade the body without being recognised and avoid attack. However, in some situations, with other predisposing factors, this goes wrong and antibodies are made, which will of course attack the body as well as the invader.

This situation has been well described in MS and RA. The bacterium *Porphyromonas gingivalis* is considered to be the main cause of periodontal disease, and it is also most frequently associated with RA. This seems to be one of the main mechanisms causing autoimmunity in RA.[5]

Autoimmune disease case study 1

A 39-year-old woman presented with joint pains of recent onset, for which she had been prescribed non-steroidal anti-inflammatory medication (NSAIDS).

She was also feeling very tired. It transpired that she had three children under eight years old and was running her own business for which she was working long hours, getting up a couple of hours before the children so she could get ahead for the day. She told me she needed to be busy.

Her digestion wasn't great, with heartburn and bloating daily.

Iridology showed lymphatic congestion and inflammation with a strong constitution.

Muscle testing indicated gluten and nightshade intolerance.

I felt that she was showing signs of possible chronic fatigue so alongside diet work, and advice to slow down, she was given a herbal prescription of:

- Reishi *Ganoderma lucidum*, an adaptogen, calming and strengthening
- Devil's claw *Harpagophytum procumbens*, an inflammation-mediating alterative
- Gotu cola *Centella asiatica*, a cooling adaptogen and inflammation mediator
- Ashwagandha *Withania somnifera*, an inflammation-mediating adaptogen.

Also a herb tea containing:

- Nettle leaf *Urtica dioica*, an inflammation-mediating alterative
- Red clover *Trifolium pretense*, an inflammation-mediating alterative targeting the lymphatic system
- Cleavers *Galium aparine*, a cooling inflammation-mediating alterative that works on the lymphatic system
- Ginger *Zingiber officinale*, a warming inflammation mediator.

I also suggested she had Epsom salts baths to help with pain.

Two weeks later blood tests gave the diagnosis of systemic lupus erythematosus (SLE), which is autoimmune in origin and was the cause of her joint pains. She wasn't able at this point to stop the NSAIDS as her joints were too painful.

It took her another year to decide to give up her business and focus on looking after herself as well as her family, and it was only when she did this that she managed to stop taking NSAIDS. She stayed on the herbs, on and off, for five years, and really learned how to care for herself, training to be a therapist so that she could put into practice what she had learned.

For more information about diet work and herbs, including a glossary, please see chapters 6 on diet and 9, the materia medica.

Autoimmune disease case study 2

A 37-year-old woman presented with Sjogren's syndrome, a condition that dries out body fluids and often results in dry itchy eyes and mouth. Sjogren's is an autoimmune disorder and is often linked with other autoimmune issues. In this case she had a lot of joint and muscle pain and fatigue, along with sinusitis, bladder irritation and always felt hot. Her acupuncturist reported that her main problem was internal fire, which fitted with all her symptoms of dried-out mucous membranes.

She had a history of tonsillitis, bladder problems and poor sleep. She also had severe premenstrual symptoms every month. She had been on methotrexate and hydroxychloroquine for four months but had now stopped these.

Muscle testing indicated dairy intolerance so she was started on a low-inflammation dairy-free diet and given a herbal tincture containing:

- Guduchi *Tinospora cordifolia*, primarily for joints, an inflammation-mediating alterative
- Marigold *Calendula officinalis*, an inflammation-mediating alterative acting on lymph and the liver
- Dandelion *Taraxacum officinale*, an alterative and bitter tonic
- Yellow dock *Rumex officinale*, an alterative and lymphatic
- Barberry *Berberis vulgaris*, an alterative and bitter tonic.

She was also advised to take a supplement formula containing magnesium and a vitamin B complex with high B6, specifically for her premenstrual syndrome, as well as vitamins C and D.

Unfortunately, within two weeks she picked up a norovirus infection, then viral meningitis, pneumonia and septicaemia; she was hospitalised for several weeks on intravenous antibiotics, steroids and analgesics.

When she finally got out of hospital she went back to her diet, plus green smoothies and probiotics. Milk thistle *Silybum marianum* was added to her herbal formula to help repair the damage done to her liver by the medications.

Muscle testing now showed salicylate sensitivity alongside the dairy intolerance, a fairly common occurrence when there is extra stress on the body. She was now quite cold and very fatigued. She was advised to drink ginger tea and a tonic formula was made for her:

• Asparagus root *Asparagus racemosus*, an inflammation-mediating, demulcent and adaptogen
• Marshmallow root *Althaea officinalis*, a vulnerary and demulcent herb
• Ashwagandha *Withania somnifera*, an inflammation-mediating adaptogen that is very helpful to improve stamina.

The next issue was oral and vaginal thrush, very likely arising from her medication while hospitalised together with her lowered immunity. So we added antifungal herbs to her first formula:

• Black walnut *Juglans nigra*
• Neem *Azadirachta indica*
• and she applied cider vinegar topically as the fungus that causes thrush, *Candida albicans*, likes an alkaline environment, so the acidification that cider vinegar creates is very effective at creating a hostile terrain for it.

Because she felt so tired all the time she felt that she needed sweet foods for energy, so these made up a lot of her diet. Sweet foods are also very comforting, but they had to be drastically reduced.

Two years after I had first seen her she returned because she was having a flare-up of her Sjogren's and had an inflamed sacroiliac joint that was giving her a lot of pain. She also said that at some point she would like to have a baby and was hoping to work towards better health so she could become pregnant.

Inflammation

We decided to put her on a gluten-free diet as well as the earlier low-salicylate and dairy-free diet. There are strong links between autoimmune disease and gluten, and she wanted to really try and regain health.

Her herbal formula was now:

- Devil's claw *Harpagophytum procumbens*, an inflammation-mediating alterative
- Ashwagandha *Withania somnifera*, an inflammation-mediating adaptogen, helpful with sleep
- Celery seed *Apium graveolens*, an inflammation-mediating alterative and digestive
- Goldenseal *Hydrastis canadensis*, a bitter mucous membrane tonic
- Angelica *Angelica archangelica*, an inflammation-mediating hepatoprotective and digestive.

She stayed on these herbs for three months and felt so much better that she decided to stop all herbs and try for a baby. Her diet remained as before. Within six weeks she was pregnant.

Her baby was induced early as she had suffered a deep vein thrombosis and had to be put on anticoagulants; she also had quite a large blood loss and a difficult delivery.

She recovered well, and the next I knew, a year later, she was expecting twins and was on heparin to prevent blood clotting. The twins were born without incident; she was doing very much better, and had learned to manage her diet and workload to moderate the major inflammatory process that was going on in her body. She had been a most dramatic patient, but was highly motivated and had come out the other end very well.

For more information about diet work and herbs, including a glossary, please see chapters 6 on diet and 9, the materia medica.

Bladder inflammation

Bladder inflammation is linked with chronic infections and irritation, most often seen with dietary factors, but also with low fluid intake. It is commonly seen with animal milk intolerance, and sometimes salicylate sensitivity, and it is usually enough to remove the irritant and use demulcent herbs such as marshmallow *Althaea officinalis*, which will heal the internal mucous membranes.

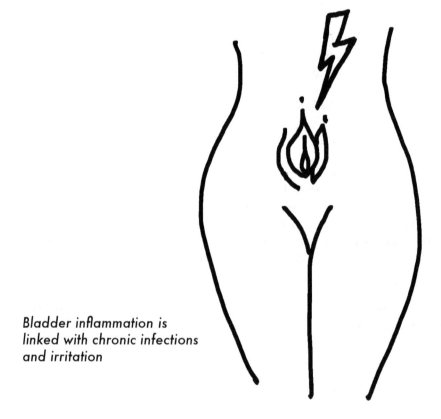

Bladder inflammation is linked with chronic infections and irritation

Bladder inflammation case study

A 54-year-old man presented with bladder irritation and frequency. His bladder was waking him at least three times every night, making sleep a real problem for him. His prostate was slightly enlarged and he had been prescribed tamsulosin, an alpha blocker that helps to relax bladder muscles. But after taking it for two months he felt it wasn't helping.

He also had digestive problems with wind, bloating and diarrhoea. He often felt hot and sweaty and said he often had very smelly sweat. He had a history of hayfever and asthma, although only used his steroid inhaler before exercise. He regularly had headaches, several times a week, for which he often took paracetamol.

On muscle testing he was found to be intolerant to dairy products. He also needed to increase his fluid intake and reduce caffeinated drinks. Alongside diet work he was given dried herbs to make a tea of which he was asked to take at least a litre a day, hot or cold.

The herbs were:

- Marshmallow leaf *Althaea officinalis*, a demulcent inflammation-mediating herb, healing to irritated mucous membranes
- Couch grass root *Agropyron repens*, a demulcent inflammation-mediating herb
- Corn silk *Zea mays*, a demulcent inflammation-mediating herb
- Wood betony *Stachys betonica*, a sedative nervine.

Within two weeks his bladder and digestion improved, and he continued with the herb tea for some years as he enjoyed drinking it. He was no longer hot and sweaty and his headaches slowly improved. He was able to stop using his inhaler after about six weeks.

For more information about diet work and herbs, including a glossary, please see chapters 6 on diet and 9, the materia medica.

Cancer

The correlation between inflammation and cancer has been known since the work of Rudolf Virchow in 1863. It is now well accepted that inflammatory mediators released during chronic inflammation promote malignant transformation of cells and carcinogenesis, as well as further development and invasiveness of malignant tumours.[6] These inflammatory mediators include TNF-alpha, IL-6, TGF-beta and IL-10, and they have been shown to participate in both the initiation and progression of cancer.[7]

Many cancers arise from sites of infection, chronic irritation and inflammation.[8] Cancer prevention therefore should focus on prevention and treatment of inflammation. When cancer has prevailed, at least part of the treatment should include diet and herbs to deal with chronic inflammation. This can easily be done alongside conventional treatment for cancer.

Cardiovascular disease

As discussed in chapter 3, the health of the endothelium is closely linked with cardiovascular disease. When there is inflammation here the result is decreased flexibility of the endothelium and raised blood pressure. Further inflammation leads to more tissue damage and then clot formation, thrombosis and stroke.

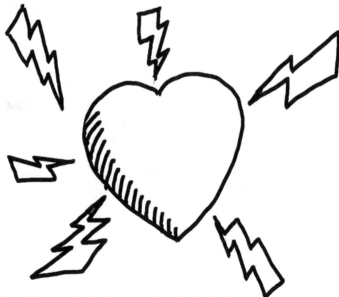

the health of the endothelium is closely linked with cardiovascular disease

Inflammation

So dealing with inflammation is the number one priority, followed by maintaining good circulation to keep everything moving. The best cardio-vascular tonic herb, hawthorn *Crataegus oxycantha*, is also inflammation-mediating and stimulates circulation among other actions.

The view that atherosclerosis is a lipid storage disease is unfortunately still prevalent, but increasingly it is being realised that inflammation is the primary issue, and that lifestyle changes can treat this better than surgery.[9,10]

A study published in 2017, which looked at risk factors for cardiovascular disease in 378,000 patients, found that the highest risk factor was chronic obstructive pulmonary disease; the second highest was when someone was taking corticosteroid medication (prescribed for an inflammatory process), and four out of the next six factors were socioeconomic. A raised LDL cholesterol featured at number 46 out of 50 risk factors – not exactly a high risk factor.[11]

Systemic inflammation is an important factor both in the development of atherosclerotic plaque and in its instability, which causes thrombotic and ischaemic events.

Chronic fatigue and fibromyalgia
Chronic fatigue, fibromyalgia, myalgic encephalitis, and probably long COVID are very similar conditions with the same basis for their symptoms. They are all based on low-grade chronic inflammation that appears to be due to an underfunctioning immune system. Initial causes will vary from one person to another but often they can be traced to a viral or other infection that hasn't resolved properly. The immune system has been overwhelmed.

This is very often also linked to stress or overwork, and the body simply goes into downtime from which it cannot be roused. The treatment will vary from person to person but it will always involve removing inflammatory foods, healing the gut, and using inflammation-mediating herbs or other treatment alongside gentle rehabilitation.

Chronic fatigue and fibromyalgia case study 1

A 17-year-old male presented with chronic fatigue syndrome, which he had been diagnosed with two years previously. He had been seeing a homeopath, which had helped a bit but he was still very tired and had digestive problems that hadn't eased.

He suffered from constant heartburn and acid reflux, as well as digestive gurgling and bubbling. He felt empty all the time so he ate more often and ended up bloated. His sleep was good, but he was often quite cold. As a small child he had been diagnosed with severe allergy to eggs and all nuts, and he carried an epipen in case he had any accidental contact with these. He had been hyperactive until the age of 13.

He had a history of severe asthma as a small child, but this was not so bad now. He had an infection in utero and had been given a seven-day course of antibiotics at birth. He regularly had tonsillitis.

His fatigue was bad enough that he could only attend school for two to three hours a day.

Muscle testing indicated the nuts and eggs, but also dairy and salicylate intolerance, which fitted with his symptom picture.

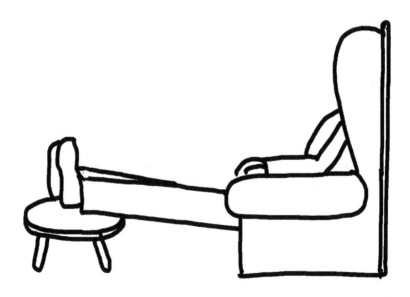

Inflammation

He was started on a low-inflammation dairy-free diet, alongside vitamin D3, magnesium and fish oils.

He was given a herbal prescription of Reishi *Ganoderma lucidum*, an adaptogen well known to be calming and strengthening, which aids sleep and is anti-allergy. This was in spore form to be used as a powder as the spores are considered the most useful format for allergic individuals.

Two month later his digestion was much better, and he had somewhat better energy levels. He still suffered from fatigue so Ashwagandha *Withania somnifera* was added to the Reishi spores as an inflammation-mediating adaptogen that is known to improve stamina.

This was helpful and he was still on these herbs three months later and steadily improving.

For more information about diet work and herbs, including a glossary, please see chapters 6 on diet and 9, the materia medica.

Chronic fatigue and fibromyalgia case study 2
A 36-year-old male had been diagnosed with fibromyalgia at the age of 25, and his muscle and joint pains had been severe enough to prevent him being active. He still had muscle and joint pains but not as severe now, although he now had digestive problems with diarrhoea and very smelly wind.

His sleep was poor, waking about 2–3am and then having difficulty going back to sleep. He had been seeing an acupuncturist, who referred him to me with their diagnosis of liver heat and spleen qi deficiency. As a child he had a history of hayfever, hives, ear infections and tonsillitis.

Muscle testing showed dairy intolerance so he was advised to eat a low-inflammation dairy-free diet. Ground linseeds were suggested to ease the diarrhoea, and he was advised to take vitamins D3 and C as well as magnesium.

He was prescribed a cooling, inflammation-mediating and digestive herbal tincture to be taken before meals:

- Sariva *Hemidesmus indicus*, an inflammation-mediating alterative and nervine

- Fennel seed *Foeniculum vulgare*, a cooling carminative and digestive
- Guduchi *Tinospora cordifolia*, primarily for joints, an inflammation-mediating alterative
- Celery seed *Apium graveolens*, an inflammation-mediating alterative and digestive
- Devil's claw *Harpagophytum procumbens*, an inflammation-mediating alterative
- Gentian *Gentiana lutea*, a cooling digestive bitter.

Three weeks later his digestion and bowels had improved, and he was sleeping better. He stayed on the herbs for another six months or so, on and off as he found it really helped with his digestion and muscle pains. He returned two years later with constant reflux and insomnia. He had been prescribed mirtazapine, an antidepressant, which improved his sleep marginally.

Muscle testing indicated that he now had an intolerance to high-salicylate foods as well as dairy, and on questioning it turned out that he had been eating some dairy products. It is very common to see salicylate sensitivity in those where there is repeated gastrointestinal damage, and this will often disappear when the gut is allowed to heal.

Two weeks after changing his diet to low-salicylate and dairy-free, he reported the reflux gone, his sleep much improved and he had stopped taking the mirtazapine.

Five years after this he turned up again with nausea and reflux. This had been severe enough that he had been multi-investigated, twice with endoscopy and also several appointments with the rheumatology clinic. It transpired that he had forgotten about the salicylate sensitivity and was drinking peppermint tea several times a day as well as taking turmeric for his joints – both of these herbs are very high in salicylates. Once he removed the high-salicylate foods from his diet everything improved very quickly again.

For more information about diet work and herbs, including a glossary, please see chapters 6 on diet and 9, the materia medica.

Inflammation

Diabetes and metabolic diseases

Metaflammation is defined as low-grade, chronic inflammation orchestrated by metabolic cells in response to excess nutrients and energy. Metabolic diseases include insulin resistance, diabetes, dyslipidaemia, cardiovascular diseases and obesity, which are all caused by and cause chronic inflammation.

When there is nutrient overload, especially when food is too high in proinflammatory fatty acids, the innate immune system is overstimulated, immune cells become unable to function properly and this results in metabolic disorders.[12]

It is estimated that one quarter of the world's adult population has metabolic syndrome,[13] affecting more than two billion people worldwide and accounting for at least three million deaths annually.[14] Metabolic syndrome is the major contributor to the increase in cardiovascular disease, which includes myocardial infarction (heart attacks) that is the main compication of atherosclerosis.

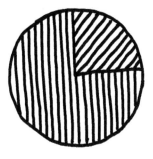

It is now recognised that fat cells, adipocytes, especially those found in abdominal fat, are able to activate, complement and produce pro-inflammatory cytokines. The links between diabetes, metabolic syndrome and inflammation are now considered to be very strong, with chronic inflammation being the root cause.[15]

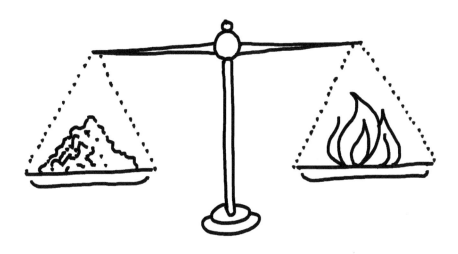

The process of inflammation leads to dysfunction of the intestinal barrier, and one study also suggests that hyperglycaemia could be the initial trigger responsible for the disruption of tight junctions.[16]

The association of dysbiosis and inflammation is also becoming apparent, linking all these processes with metabolic syndrome.[17]

There is also a bidirectional connection with oral dysbiosis, periodontal disease and diabetes. When periodontal disease is treated, HbA1c and inflammatory markers reduce significantly.[18]

A strong link between severe illness due to COVID-19 and metabolic disease has been shown. A study of over 900,000 hospitalisations in the USA up to November 2020 showed that 64% of those hospitalised were obese, had diabetes, hypertension and/or heart failure.[19]

Poorly controlled blood sugar has been shown to increase the risk of developing Alzheimer's disease, which has been termed diabetes type 3 as the brain becomes insulin resistant, which makes it unable to function properly. The links between diabetes and Alzheimer's disease seem to be very strong.[20]

Two herbs that have shown the ability to increase insulin sensitivity and also to reduce inflammation are nettle *Urtica dioica* and milk thistle *Silybum marianum*. In just eight weeks HbA1c was reduced by an average of 1.2% (7.3 down to 6.1) and there was a significant reduction in C reactive protein (CRP). This was on a dose of 3ml three times a day of a nettle tincture, without any dietary changes. This was quite amazing and could have been even more amazing with dietary changes. Nettle leaf tea could very likely have the same effect.[21]

Milk thistle was found to have an inflammation-mediating effect on the liver and also to reduce HbA1C by 1.92%. Fenugreek *Trigonella foenum-graecum* was also found to have similar effects on HbA1C.[22]

There are several other herbs useful for helping control blood sugar levels. These include gurmar *Gymnema sylvestre*, andrographis *Andrographis paniculata*, burdock root *Arctium lappa*, elderberry *Sambucus nigra*, and aniseed *Pimpinella anisum*.

More information on these herbs can be found in chapter 9, the materia medica.

Diabetes and metabolic diseases case study

A woman aged 62 presented as a longstanding type 2 diabetic on insulin and metformin. She came to see me because she had experienced a severe viral infection some months earlier for which she had required both antibiotics and steroid medication. This had resulted in her finding food a problem so she had changed her diet significantly, focusing on juices, smoothies and soups as eating had become difficult.

The result of this new diet, however, was that her blood sugar had become much more stable and she had been able to reduce her requirement for insulin and metformin blood sugar medication by about half. She wanted more advice about diet and diabetes as she had received none from the National Health Service. Her other issue was overactive bowels – she needed to defecate up to twenty times a day and often three or four times a night. She also had osteoarthritis, itchy skin and hayfever, all of which were longstanding issues. So she had inflammation going on in her digestive tract, joints, respiratory tract and skin.

Muscle testing indicated dairy and salicylate sensitivity, and she was eating far too much fruit, which is often high in salicylates and sugar.

She was started on a low-inflammation dairy-free and low-salicylate diet as well as a powder formula to help with digestive inflammation:

- Slippery elm inner bark *Ulmus fulva*, a vulnerary and demulcent herb
- Marshmallow root *Althaea officinalis*, a vulnerary and demulcent herb
- Cardamom *Elettaria cardamomum*, a carminative digestive herb.

She was also advised to take ground linseeds to help with diarrhoea. Advice was given regarding the best foods to keep blood sugar balanced through the day; and emphasis was placed on the need for her to closely monitor her blood sugar and insulin requirements as this was likely to change with her new diet.

Three weeks later she returned to say that her bowels were much less explosive and frequent, and everything was slowly improving.

Her herbal formula was changed to one more focused on inflammation and blood sugar management:

- Guduchi *Tinospora cordifolia*, primarily for joints, an inflammation-mediating alterative
- Fenugreek *Trigonella foenum-graecum*, an inflammation-mediating carminative and hypoglycaemic
- Gymnema *Gymnema sylvestre*, an inflammation-mediating hypoglycaemic
- Turmeric *Curcuma longa*, an inflammation-mediating alterative
- Black pepper *Piper nigrum*, a carminative that improves absorption of turmeric.

She was advised to take probiotics or fermented foods to improve her bowel flora.

She stayed on this herbal formula for about six months, during which time she was able to stop all insulin and metformin, and her blood sugar became very stable.

At her request she then started taking Reishi mushroom *Ganoderma lucidum*, an adaptogen that can be taken long term and has has been shown to have excellent stabilising properties in diabetes. This she stayed on for several years and found it to be very effective.

For more information about diet work and herbs, including a glossary, please see chapters 6 on diet and 9, the materia medica.

Inflammatory and irritable gut diseases

Inflammatory gut or bowel diseases (IBD) include Crohn's disease and ulcerative colitis, both very debilitating conditions that involve frequent and bloody diarrhoea, malabsorption and pain. The incidence of these is increasing, for reasons that include antibiotic use, medications such as non-steroidal anti-inflammatories, oral contraceptives and air pollution.[23]

With many IBD, symptoms appear in the mouth first as ulcers, glossitis, periodontal disease or angular cheilitis. There is a strong link between oral dysbiosis, periodontal disease and later-onset IBD.

All these factors have their long-term effect as inflammation, and together with dietary and lifestyle causes of inflammation can be reasonably given as underlying reasons for IBD. Treating IBD involves dietary changes and the use of herbs to mediate inflammation and heal the digestive system.

See chapter 3 on how to improve gut health.

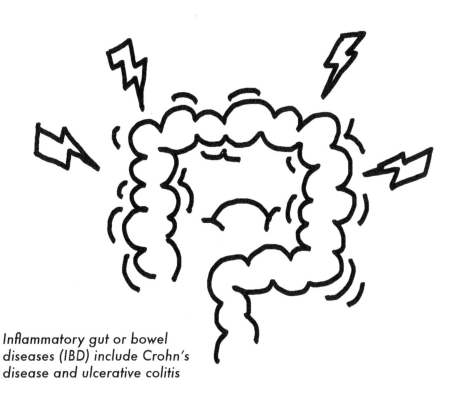

Inflammatory gut or bowel diseases (IBD) include Crohn's disease and ulcerative colitis

Inflammatory and irritable gut diseases case study

A 47-year-old woman presented with inflammatory bowel disease, probably ulcerative colitis. It was not severe but she had experienced some gastrointestinal bleeding for which she had been prescribed mesalazine, an aminosalicylate drug that acts as anti-inflammatory to the digestive system. This had been going on for some years, and had always improved when she was pregnant.

She had two children, aged 8 and 9, and had also suffered several miscarriages. She had a history of cystitis and regularly had to get up twice a night to urinate. Her sleep wasn't very good as she found it difficult to go back to sleep.

She also had pityriasis in her scalp. She had a great deal of stress in her life, made worse because she was a perfectionist and felt she was the only person keeping the family going.

Iridology showed a great deal of inflammation in a very strong constitution. Muscle testing indicated dairy and salicylate sensitivity.

She was put on a low-inflammation, low-salicylate and dairy-free diet.

Ginger tea was suggested as she was very often cold, and this treatment would be warming as well as inflammation-mediating.

She was prescribed slippery elm *Ulmus fulva* and marshmallow root *Althaea officinalis* powders to be taken before meals, and L-glutamine powder, also to be taken before meals. Slippery elm and marshmallow root are both excellent vulnerary and demulcent herbs as well as acting as prebiotics. L-glutamine is a supplement useful in healing badly damaged gastrointestinal systems.

She missed her next appointment and finally returned a year later with worse symptoms than before. Her diet had gone awry (her words) and she was now bleeding again with diarrhoea and abdominal cramping, and severe fatigue. She had restarted her diet two weeks previously and said there had already been some improvement, but she was concerned about the level of fatigue she was experiencing.

She had recently had blood tests done and was not anaemic. She was still experiencing stress and was now homeschooling her children so life was very full on.

I suggested a multivitamin might be useful, alongside extra magnesium and vitamin C, as she was probably malabsorbing. She was to stay on L-glutamine, slippery elm and marshmallow root, plus ginger tea.

Her herbal formula was a tincture comprised of:

- Vervain *Verbena officinalis*, a nervine bitter
- Wild yam *Dioscorea villosa*, an antispasmodic inflammation-mediating adrenal tonic
- Agrimony *Agrimonia eupatoria*, an inflammation-mediating, astringent digestive tonic
- Blessed thistle *Cnicus benedictus*, a nervine antispasmodic digestive bitter
- Goldenseal *Hydrastis Canadensis*, a mucous membrane bitter tonic
- Ginger *Zingiber officinale*, a warming inflammation-mediating digestive.

This formula was to be taken in drop doses before meals to help digestion, and could also be used if she had any cramping pains.

Again I didn't see her for another year, and the next I heard was that she was now in hospital with severe ulcerative colitis. Her doctors wanted to start her on azathioprine, an immunosuppressant medication with fairly difficult potential side effects. She really didn't want to take this so was asking for help again.

Again her diet had slipped so she knew what she had to do. This time she managed to stick to it, and with the help of the herbs prescribed previously, and her family's support she managed to have a good outcome. At least that was the last I heard.

For more information about diet work and herbs, including a glossary, please see chapters 6 on diet and 9, the materia medica.

Inflammatory lung diseases

Chronic inflammatory diseases in the lungs are usually caused by pathogenic microorganisms or by toxins, pollutants, allergens or other irritants. Disease states include asthma, bronchiectasis, chronic bronchitis, emphysema and pulmonary fibrosis. Causes vary from microbial infection to smoking and smoke inhalation from cooking stoves.

The first line of defence in the lungs are the epithelial cells lining the airway. This is non-specific immunity, the barrier function, and the epithelial cells secrete defensive chemicals such as mucins, lysozyme and nitric oxide that protect against microorganisms. They also secrete inflammatory mediators such as reactive oxygen radicals, cytokines (including TNF-alpha) and platelet activating factor to attract macrophages and other inflammatory cells to the site.[24]

Immunological responses follow as the specific immunity comes into play with lymphocytes and antibody response.

Sometimes in chronic inflammatory lung conditions there is no proper resolution because the causative factor is not removed, and also because the lung tissue can be so damaged that it can't mount a proper immune response. Mucus formation is excessive and can become thick and stagnant, creating a situation where more infections can proliferate.

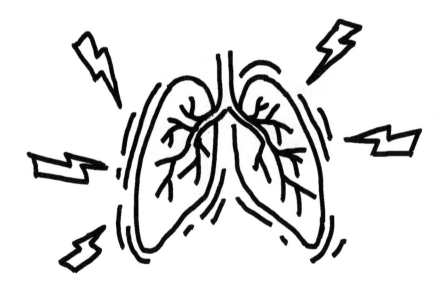

Inflammation

Inflammatory lung diseases case study 1

A 68-year-old woman presented with a long history of bronchiectasis, where long-term damage to the lungs leaves the airways abnormally wide, making them highly vulnerable to infection. She had a long history of chest infections, tonsillitis and sinusitis. She wanted to avoid the flu vaccination as, when she had received it the year before, she had been very ill. So she felt she really needed to improve her lung health.

She was otherwise an active and busy woman. She was already taking probiotics, which she did fairly regularly because she very often had to take antibiotics.

Muscle testing indicated dairy intolerance so she was started on a low-inflammation dairy-free diet. Ginger tea was advised as a good anti-inflammatory herb that should also help to keep her lungs clear of excess mucus. She needed expectorant herbs as well as lung-restorative and inflammation-medicating herbs.

Her prescription was:

- Thyme *Thymus vulgaris*, an inflammation-mediating lung tonic and antimicrobial
- Holy basil *Ocimum sanctum*, an inflammation-mediating vulnerary and adaptogen acting particularly on the lungs
- Elecampane *Inula helenium*, an antitussive bronchodilator and lung tonic
- White horehound *Marrubium vulgare*, an antispasmodic expectorant
- Echinacea *Echinacea purpurea*, an inflammation-mediating immunostimulant
- Yerba mansa *Anemopsis californica*, an astringent bitter with antifungal and antibacterial properties
- *Lobelia inflata*, an antispasmodic targeting the respiratory tract.

She also had a bottle of *Eucalyptus radiata* essential oil to use as a steam inhalation to help both lungs and sinuses. This proved very helpful and she stayed on this formula for some time.

Two years later she had a cold, which led to a chest infection and sinus congestion. She had antibiotics and went back on the herbal formula again. This time a few drops of essential oil of *Thymus mastichina* was added to her tincture as a stronger antimicrobial. This is safe if used in the correct dilution, but should not be attempted without proper knowl-

The results of inflammation

edge. She was in some pain from the sinus congestion so she was given a nasal spray containing *Anemopsis californica* and *Hydrastis canadensis*, a combination that is very good at clearing stubborn sinus infections.

Over the years she came back from time to time, especially if she thought she might be starting a chest infection. Most times she managed to avoid using antibiotics. Various herbs were used depending on her main symptoms. Two herbs in particular were helpful:

- Ground ivy *Glechoma hederacea*, an inflammation-mediating decongestant, expectorant, antihistamine and antimicrobial
- Goldenrod *Solidago virgaurea*, an inflammation-mediating decongestant.

About five years after her first visit she was told she had hypertension, and she very much wanted to avoid medication. She had the feeling of a tight band around her chest and could feel her heartbeat. She also had a lot of stress in her life at this point.

Her herbal tincture was:

- Hawthorn *Crataegus monogyna, C. oxyacantha*, an inflammation-mediating cardiotonic and nervine
- Cactus *Selenicereus grandiflora*, a cardiotonic and nervine specific for feelings of a tight band around chest
- Motherwort *Leonurus cardiac*, a cardiotonic, hypotensive and nervine
- Mistletoe *Viscum alba*, a nervine, hypotensive and vasodilator
- Reishi *Ganoderma lucidum*, a sedative adaptogen, hypotensive and inflammation-mediating.

She had this formula with some variations for most of the next five years. It kept her blood pressure under control as long as she didn't get too stressed. During this time she found she needed her lung herbs less often; very slowly her lungs seemed to be healing and she had fewer incidences of chest infections.

For more information about diet work and herbs, including a glossary, please see chapters 6 on diet and 9, the materia medica.

Inflammatory lung diseases case study 2
A 58-year-old woman presented with poor sleep and asthma. She took

a long time to fall asleep, sometimes several hours, and then woke at 4am, unable to get back to sleep again. She also had digestive discomfort with wind and bloating, and very often felt hot, which she thought was not menopausal. She was taking several medications for asthma, including a preventer (beclomethasone), a treater (salbutamol) and an extra bronchodilator (serevent) as well as nasal drops for postnasal drip. She had a long history of sinus congestion. She was keen to come off her medication.

Muscle testing indicated dairy and soya intolerance, so she was started on an anti-inflammatory diet without dairy or soya. She was advised to take holy basil *Ocimum sanctum* as a tea.

Her herbal formula was a tincture comprised of:

- Coriander *Coriandrum sativum*, a cooling digestive and decongestant
- Yerba mansa *Anemopsis californica*, a cooling bitter decongestant alterative
- Goldenrod *Solidago virgaurea*, an inflammation-mediating decongestant and vulnerary
- Wood betony *Stachys betonica*, a nervine bitter tonic
- Reishi *Ganoderma lucidum*, an adaptogen that calms and strengthens, aids sleep and is anti-allergy.

She was also given a small bottle of lobelia *Lobelia inflata*, an antispasmodic targeting the respiratory tract. This was to be used as needed to replace the treater inhaler when possible.

Within one month her sleep had improved a great deal, and she no longer needed the nasal drops or the salbutamol inhaler. Her sinuses were also improving. She enjoyed the holy basil tea very much.

She stayed on the tincture and lobelia for over a year during which time she slowly stopped all her medication. Over the next two years she reduced the herbs until she just used lobelia very occasionally with holy basil tea, and this, together with a dairy- and soya-free diet, was all she needed.

For more information about diet work and herbs, including a glossary, please see chapters 6 on diet and 9, the materia medica.

Inflammatory skin diseases

The chronic inflammatory skin diseases include psoriasis, eczema and acne. Conventionally these are defined by descriptive assessment. These are all inflammatory, influenced by the gut microbiome,[25] and also often autoimmune too.

The skin is our largest organ of elimination, and also has its own microbiome of commensal bacteria that protect the skin. In these days of excessive daily washing, soaps and disinfectants the skin flora often suffers, but all inflammatory skin diseases need treating from the inside, usually starting with the gut.

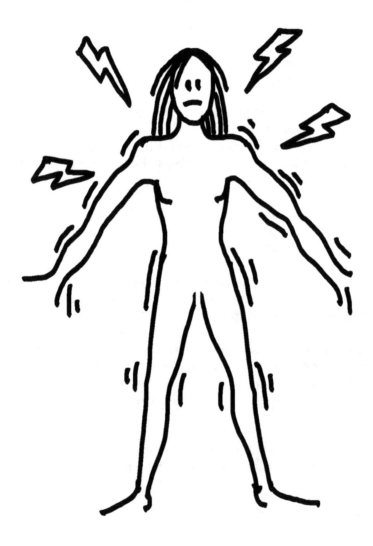

Inflammatory skin disease case study

A woman aged 37 presented with eczema for which she had been pre-scribed a steroid cream. She was having night sweats but had no signs of early menopause. She had experienced eczema as a child, but it had dis-appeared until three years previously and was now very hot and itchy, all over her body, and really quite severe.

She had a history of cystitis, and had experienced it four times in the last year, each time taking antibiotics for five days. Her sleep was very poor because of the itching and heat. She also had a history of tonsillitis and ear infections as a child, for which she had taken a lot of antibiotics.

Unsurprisingly, testing showed she was intolerant to dairy products, but also to high-salicylate foods. Alongside a low-inflammatory diet, fermented foods to replace her gut flora, no dairy and a low-salicylate diet she was started on herbs to cool her and treat her skin. Removing the inflammatory foods was the most important change but alterative herbs to improve lymph and liver function as well as all elimination systems were also indicated.

Her herbal prescription was a tea of:

- Heartsease *Viola tricolor*, a cooling inflammation-mediating alterative
- Cleavers *Galium aparine*, a cooling inflammation-mediating alterative that targets the lymphatic system.

She also had a tincture of:

- Oregon grape *Mahonia aquifolium*, an alterative targeting the liver and digestive system
- Dandelion root *Taraxacum officinale*, an alterative targeting the liver and digestive system, also a diuretic to improve elimination
- Vervain *Verbena officinalis*, a cooling alterative and nervine
- Gotu cola *Hydrocotyle asiatica*, a cooling adaptogen and inflamma-tion-mediator that is useful for skin problems.

When treating skin diseases it is vital to improve elimination systems in order to provide an exit from the body for the toxins that have caused the skin problems.

Over the next six weeks her sleep and heat improved quite quickly. Her skin took a bit longer but did finally improve. She only needed the herbs for three months in total.

Three years later she had a flare-up after the death of her mother; a repeat of the herbal prescriptions and a reminder of the diet work improved things quite quickly.

For more information about diet work and herbs, including a glossary, please see chapters 6 on diet and 9, the materia medica.

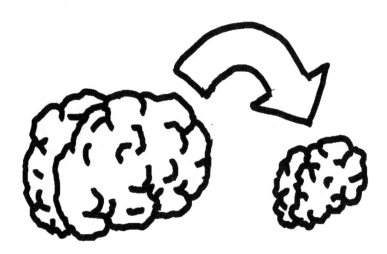

Neurodegenerative disease
Neurodegenerative disease covers a range of conditions that affect the neurons in the brain. As neurons are not normally replaced, once damaged by inflammation the effect on the brain is either ataxia (impaired movement) or dementia (impaired mental function). Examples of neurodegenerative disease include Alzheimer's disease, motor neurone disease, Parkinson's disease and Huntington's disease.

These diseases derive from inflammation that alters proteins in the brain, which then form different structures that aggregate and become toxic to other brain cells. In Alzheimer's disease these structures are amyloid plaques and tau tangles.[26]

Inflammation

It appears that the amyloid plaques may be part of the body's defence mechanism, a process that attempts to protect the brain against inflammation. This was shown by an experiment where an amyloid-directed monoclonal antibody actually removed plaques in people with Alzheimer's disease, but no clinical improvement followed.[27]

There are definite links between the gut microbiome and neuroinflammation in most neurodegenerative diseases.

Neuroinflammation is the body's response to injury or infection of the nervous system. There is a two-way communication between the gastrointestinal tract and the central nervous system known as the gut microbiota–brain axis, and this signals the brain to mount an immune response, which becomes chronic and out of control. The initial neuroprotective process becomes neurotoxic.[28]

There also appears to be another source of inflammation affecting the brain from endotoxins, the lipopolysaccharides (LPS) present in the membrane of gram negative bacteria. These are increased in dysbiosis, and bacterial infection including periodontitis and when the bacteria die off and there is a degree of gut leakiness. Then the released LPS can move through the intestinal wall and into the bloodstream where they will initiate inflammation.

Endotoxins damage neurons by activating the inflammatory process in the brain that promotes amyloid plaques and tau aggregation tangles.[29]

One study showed that for people with Alzheimer's disease, those with the most brain plaque also had the highest levels of inflammation and LPS.[30]

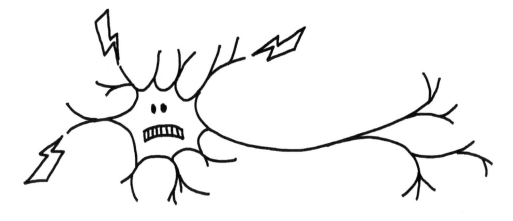

Porphyromonas gingivalis, the main pathogenic bacteria involved in periodontitis, has actually been found in the brains of those with Alzheimer's disease. *P. gingivalis* has been shown to produce toxic enzymes that affect brain tissue. Antibodies against *P. gingivalis* have been found in the brains of many of those with Alzheimer's.

All these factors have been shown to create the amyloid beta and plaque lesions of Alzheimer's disease.[31]

Viral infections have long been suspected to be an underlying cause for neuroinflammatory diseases, although this has been hard to prove. Certainly viral infections can trigger autoimmune disease, for example a variant of herpes simplex can result in autoimmune encephalitis, which will continue even if the virus is treated. This has been seen in many people infected by SARS-CoV-2 who continue to suffer multiple neurological symptoms such as cognitive dysfunction, pain and fatigue, and more severe neuroimmune disorders such as encephalomyelitis or acute necrotising haemorrhagic encephalopathy (ANE).[32]

Diets and lifestyles that result in reduced inflammation have shown good results with neurodegenerative diseases, examples being the Bredesen protocol[33] and the MIND diet, a hybrid of the Mediterranean diet and the dietary approaches to stop hypertension, which have both been associated with a slower cognitive decline and lower risk of Alzheimer's disease dementia in older adults.[34]

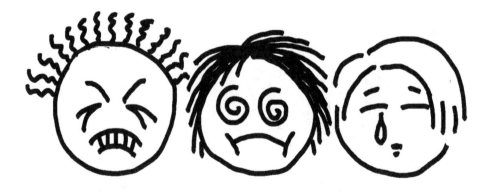

Inflammation is frequently named as the root cause of all psychiatric conditions

Inflammation

Mental health problems

This is a quote from a professor of psychiatry in the USA:

"When I attended medical school in the mid-1980s, no one imagined that the immune system had anything to do with the brain. When I became a researcher in 2000, we were convinced that inflammation would only be relevant to patients with medical illnesses that might account for their immune activation. Now, in 2018 I find myself amazed that inflammation is frequently named as the root cause of all psychiatric conditions – the sine qua non of all mental illness."[35]

Any stress creates an inflammatory process in the body, so all mental health problems will have stress associated with them, but it is far from the only underlying cause of mental health problems. So, for example, depression can be caused by inflammation, but it is not only caused by inflammation.[36]

As ever, if diet is involved in reducing inflammation, there is a beneficial result on mental health. There is also a beneficial effect on the microbiome, which interacts with the brain using neural, inflammatory and hormonal signalling pathways, resulting in benefits to mental health.[37]

Mental health problems case study

A young man aged 25 had been suffering with anxiety and depression for eight years. He had tried cognitive behavioural therapy, counselling and hypnosis as well as taking fluoxetine, but he felt that nothing had really helped. He was also experiencing fatigue, especially after eating. His sleep was disturbed and he woke in the morning feeling unrefreshed. He had a history of ear infections, tonsillitis and sinusitis from childhood onwards.

His diet was very high in sugar, with several teaspoons of sugar in his many cups of tea every day as well as cordial drinks, and also he ate a lot of refined white wheat products such as pasta and white bread, biscuits and cakes.

Muscle testing indicated dairy intolerance, which fitted with his medical history, so he started on a dairy-free low-inflammation diet.

He was given flower essences to help his anxiety and depression, specifically the Bach remedies star of Bethlehem (for shock), mimulus (for fear), sweet chestnut (for extreme mental anguish) and also echinacea flower essence, which is a fundamental remedy for self-esteem and for those feeling as though they are falling apart.

It was also suggested that he should take probiotics or fermented foods to improve his microbiome.

Six weeks later he reported feeling like a new person, ready to start reducing his fluoxetine and eventually stop it completely. This was a case of a young man whose inflammation was coming solely from his diet, and because he was still young and inflammation wasn't too entrenched, simply changing his diet was enough to deal with it. The flower remedies are very useful to buy time and give a boost to emotions while doing the, sometimes difficult, task of changing one's diet.

For more information about diet work and herbs, including a glossary, please see chapters 6 on diet and 9, the materia medica.

Osteoporosis
Osteoporosis is very often seen alongside autoimmune inflammatory conditions such as rheumatoid arthritis, systemic lupus erythematosus and ankylosing spondylitis.[38]

Studies have shown systemic bone loss throughout the body alongside systemic inflammation, whereas localised inflammation is linked with localised bone loss. There is an interaction between bone and the immune system cells that has an effect on bone mineralisation and resorption, resulting in bone loss when there is inflammation because osteoclast activity (bone resorption) is favoured over osteoblast activity (bone formation).

The level of C-reactive protein was also found to be associated with bone mineral density.[39]

Chronic pain
Chronic pain is a part of most of the above chronic diseases, and is a very common problem affecting millions of people. It might include headaches, migraines, cancer pain, joint pain, muscle pain or nerve pain. The underlying causes will vary a lot, but the pain is usually due to inflammation affecting the local nerves, sending messages via the spinal cord to the brain.

Treating pain is therefore about treating the underlying cause of the inflammation. There are some herbs that will also treat the actual pain itself.

They are not as strong as pain-relieving medications but are also not as risky. These might include frankincense *Boswellia serrata*, feverfew *Tanacetum parthenium*, corydalis *Corydalis* spp. and cannabis *Cannabis sativa*.

Castor oil packs are excellent at moving stagnation in tissues, which is also a cause of pain, and can be used over a painful area with some success. I have successfully prescribed castor oil packs for the bone pain of cancer, and painful livers in chronic liver diseases.

Chapter summary:
The chronic inflammatory diseases include the following list, which are described from a holistic point of view, and some have case studies:

- allergies
- arthritis
- autoimmune diseases
- bladder inflammation
- cancer
- cardiovascular disease
- chronic fatigue and fibromyalgia
- diabetes and metabolic diseases
- inflammatory and irritable gut diseases
- inflammatory lung diseases
- inflammatory skin diseases
- neurodegenerative disease
- mental health problems
- osteoporosis
- chronic pain.

6
Using diet to reduce inflammation

Getting the diet right is probably the most important step in combating chronic inflammation.

There is no single diet that will be right for everyone but there are some factors that are common to all:

- A large variety of plant-based foods is vital for everyone, because they contain a wide range of phytonutrients (see below), minerals and vitamins. While five a day might be adequate, ten a day is a far better target. Most plant foods should be vegetables rather than fruit, because of fruit's high sugar content.

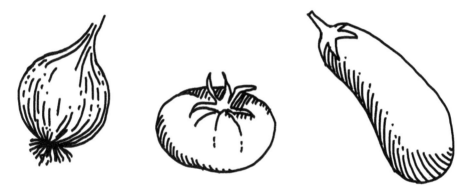

- Unprocessed natural foods are better for the body than processed foods. That means wholegrains rather than refined grains.
- Oils and fats can be pro-inflammatory or anti-inflammatory, and choosing the best ones is important as good oils and fats are vital for health. See below for more information.
- Some foods are inflammatory to everyone. These include sugar, especially that derived from corn; gluten grains (wheat, rye, barley and sometimes oats); animal milk products; oranges; pork meat, and especially processed and preserved pork products such as bacon and sausages; alcohol; and trans fats (see below). Foods with a high glycaemic index are generally pro-inflammatory.[1]
- Fructose appears to be even more inflammatory than glucose. Fructose has been shown to contribute to metabolic disease, to increase cytokine production and inflammation independent of metabolic disease.[2]

- Other foods are inflammatory to individuals only if they are intolerant or allergic to them. These might include gluten, eggs, nuts, seeds, soya, and nightshade family foods. These are the immunological intolerances and allergies, known as immunological because they create antibodies and hence a memory in the body that will react whenever that food enters the body.
- There are also foods that seem to be more irritant, and that cause a problem when there is already gut damage. These include gluten and the high-salicylate foods such as berries, turmeric and cinnamon.
- Weight loss where someone is overweight is always going to reduce inflammation.[3]

Food intolerances
These can be immunological or they can be irritant. The latter usually only cause a problem if the former are already present and have damaged gut tissue so that it is vulnerable.

Immunological intolerances are not outgrown. If they affect a child or baby they will still be present when that child grows up. The manifestation of the intolerance can change, though, so that it appears that they are outgrown.

In children and babies the manifestation of a food intolerance is likely to be obvious and often acute, and vomiting, diarrhoea and skin rashes are all commonly seen. In adults these symptoms tend to internalize, so they become irritable bowel syndrome, which is managed and coped with, or atherosclerosis, which is silent until it becomes a problem. Or they might be arthritic joint changes that are slow to manifest. In other words, silent inflammation that creeps in unannounced.

Some peptides in foods are identical to peptides in body tissue. For example, wheat contains some identical peptides to those present in collagen. So if there is an immunological reaction to a food, creating antibodies against that food, those antibodies will also attack the body tissue. This is called molecular mimicry.

Cross-reactive peptides have been identified in milk, corn, soya, eggs and some nuts.

Molecular mimicry is found between various infective microorganisms and human tissue. The idea is that the microorganism can invade the body without being recognised and avoid attack. However, in some situations, with other predisposing factors, this goes wrong and antibodies are made

Inflammation

that will attack the body as well as the invader. This situation has been well described in multiple sclerosis (MS), and in rheumatoid arthritis (RA), and is one of the main mechanisms causing autoimmunity.[4]

Irritant foods
These cause damage and irritation when there is already some gut damage. The foods concerned include the gliadin peptides in gluten, which is found in the gluten grains, wheat, rye, oats and barley. These cereals have been shown to cause inflammation in the intestinal wall by non-immunological means, that is, without antibody formation. They damage the villi, the protruding fingers of the intestinal wall, and can induce leaky gut as well as inflammation.

This, together with molecular mimicry and probably viral infections, are the most probable underlying causes of coeliac disease, an autoimmune condition whereby gluten damages the intestinal villi, causing malabsorption, diarrhoea and bleeding.[5]

Non-coeliac gluten sensitivity is possibly more common than coeliac gluten sensitivity, and as well as the digestive symptoms, other common indicators include fatigue, joint and muscle pain, headaches and brain fog. For anyone with autoimmune disease in particular, but also anyone with chronic inflammation that doesn't improve, it is important to at least try eliminating gluten for a few months to see what difference it makes.

In some cases, the irritant in grains is the weedkiller glyphosate, which is used almost routinely to kill off non-organic grain crops so they are dry enough to be harvested. Glyphosate acts as an antibiotic and was considered to be safe for human (and animal) consumption, but it is now known that it slowly destroys the microbiome, causing inflammation and chronic ill health.[6] Glyphosate residues have been found in most non-organic grain-based cereals, and in many samples of wheat and oats.

High-salicylate foods are less damaging than gluten but can cause a great deal of irritation in those who become sensitive to them. Examples of high-salicylate foods include all the berries, especially strawberries, chamomile, liquorice, cinnamon and turmeric. Certainly there has been an increase in salicylate sensitivity, especially in those who have been taking high doses of turmeric for inflammatory disease. In this situation turmeric will actually make things worse. My usual recommendation for turmeric, which is a useful inflammation-mediating herb, is not to take it every day.

For more information on high-salicylate foods and herbs please see p. 126.

Foods containing high amounts of lectins can cause problems for some people, especially if they already have some gut damage. Many foods contain lectins as they are plant chemicals designed to protect seeds as they pass through the digestive tract, so they are still viable when they emerge at the other end. So lectins are not digested, although they can provoke an immune response as they pass through. Gluten is a lectin. Most lectins are destroyed by soaking, cooking and/or sprouting, and as most high-lectin foods tend to be prepared for eating in this manner, in general they are not so much of a problem.

High-lectin foods include most grains and legumes, so that means wheat, rice, barley, quinoa, soya, lentils, kidney beans and chickpeas. In this group of foods, lectins are greatly reduced by adequate soaking, cooking or sprouting. Undercooked legumes are difficult to digest, and cause a reaction, which can be severe, in many people.

Other high-lectin foods include sunflower and pumpkin seeds, cashews, peanuts and the nightshade family group (tomatoes, aubergines, potatoes, chillies, sweet peppers), and also cucumbers. Lectins are greatly reduced in cucumbers and nightshades when they are peeled and deseeded.

Phytonutrients
Phytonutrients are naturally occurring chemicals found in plants that are used for the plant's defence and welfare. They are also often very helpful for human health, which is why we need a wide variety of plant-based foods in our diets.

Phytonutrients all have different properties but in general protect tissue cells from damage, and help repair damage when it does occur. Many of them regulate the inflammatory response and are antioxidants. Several hundred thousand different phytonutrients have been identified in various plant foods, and some of these are well-researched and understood.

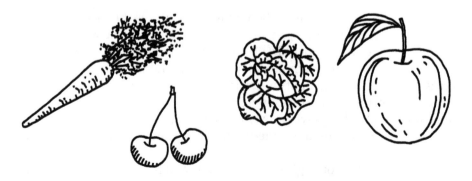

These include:

- Carotenoids: more than 600 different carotenoids provide the yellow, orange and red colours in fruit, vegetables and herbs; all are excellent antioxidants. They include beta-carotene, an antioxidant found in carrots – alpha carotene and beta-carotene are converted by the body into vitamin A – lutein and zeaxanthin, which are found in egg yolks, spinach and kale, and protect the eyes from cataracts and macular degeneration; and lycopene, which is found in tomatoes and watermelon and is an important protective against heart disease and prostate cancer.
- Flavonoids: these include catechins from green tea that are protective against cancer; hesperidin from citrus fruit that reduces inflammation; and flavonols from apples, berries, kale and onions that reduce asthma and cardiovascular disease.
- Resveratrol is a powerful antioxidant found in red grape skins, and hence red wine, which is associated with reduced risk of cardiovascular disease.
- Glucosinolates are derived from cruciferous vegetables such as broccoli, cabbage and kale, and have been shown to reduce the risk of cancer, cardiovascular disease and inflammation generally.
- Ellagic acid is found in red berries and pomegranates, and is another good antioxidant able to protect against inflammation and cancer.
- Anthocyanins are found in purple foods such as blueberries, blackcurrants and red cabbage, and are excellent antioxidants with benefits in cancer, cardiovascular disease, diabetes and eyesight.

It is often suggested that to get all these amazing phytonutrients in the diet the best way is to 'eat a rainbow'. This means making sure there are foods of all colours eaten throughout the day, with a good variety of colours at every meal. It is possible to taste the difference between foods containing good amounts of phytonutrients and those without: the ripest, healthiest fruit and vegetables will have the best flavour and will contain the most phytonutrients.

Oils for cooking and eating

Choosing the healthiest option when it comes to fats and oils is an area fraught with disagreement, myths and misinformation. There is now no doubt that a low-fat diet is not the healthiest option for most people, and it is not the best anti-inflammatory diet. We need the right fats and oils in our diet to be healthy.

Good fats and oils are important for several reasons:

- Vitamins A, D, E and K are fat-soluble, which means they can only be absorbed from the diet if accompanied by fats.
- The omega-3 fatty acids eicoosapentaenoic acid (EPA) and docosahexaenoic acid (DHA) are essential as anti-inflammatories, for brain, nervous system and eye health, and cannot be made in the body.
- Cell growth and wound healing require fats and essential fatty acids.

There are four kinds of fats in the diet, depending on the proportion and type of the fatty acids that make them up:

- Saturated fats are those that are solid at room temperature; these are often, but not only, animal-based. Examples are butter, beef or pork dripping, and coconut oil.
- Polyunsaturated and monounsaturated fats are liquid at room temperature and are rich in essential fatty acids, omega 3, 6, 9 and 12. These tend to be plant-based oils and fats. Examples are sunflower, olive, hemp seed and walnut oils.
- Trans fats are a processed form of fats formed when vegetable oil is solidified in a process called hydrogenation, so that it doesn't go rancid so quickly. Trans fats are found in margarines and in many processed foods because they act as a preservative. These are widely understood to be very unhealthy, as they increase the 'bad' cholesterol, LDL, and reduce the 'good' cholesterol, HDL.

Contrary to the advice that has been offered for many years, there is no association between the intake of saturated fats, monounsaturated fats or polyunsaturated fats and risk of cardiovascular disease (CVD).

The idea that saturated fat clogs an artery like a pipe is wrong. However, there is a greater risk of CVD and all-cause mortality with a higher intake of trans fats; as well as a cardioprotective effect from polyunsaturated fats.[7]

There is no association between saturated fat consumption and mortality, cardiovascular disease, stroke or diabetes. In the prevention

Inflammation

of cardiovascular disease there is no benefit from reduced fat, including saturated fat.[8,9]

Oils also vary in their smoke point, in other words, in the temperature at which they burn and become injurious to health. Oils with a high smoke point are fine for cooking with, whereas those with a low smoke point are not. The accompanying table gives some ideas as to which oils and fats are healthiest from these aspects.

	SFA %	MUFA %	PUFA %	Omega 3 %	Omega 6 %	Ratio 6:3	Smoke point
Avocado oil	11	70	13	1	12	13:1	+++
Beef dripping	50	42	4	<1	3	5:1	+++
Butter	63	26	4	<1	3	7:1	++
Clarified butter	62	29	4	1	2	1:1	+++
Coconut oil	83	6	2	<1	2	88:1	++
Corn oil	13	28	55	1	53	46:1	+++
Flaxseed oil	9	18	68	53	14	1:3.7	+
Hemp seed oil	11	14	75	17	57	3.3:1	++
Lard (pig fat)	39	45	11	1	10	10:1	++
Olive oil	14	73	11	<1	9	13:1	++
Pumpkin seed oil	20	25	55	<1	55	127:1	++
Rapeseed oil	7	63	28	9	18	2:1	+++
Sesame oil	14	40	41	<1	41	137:1	+++
Sunflower oil	10	45	40	<1	40	199:1	+++
Walnut oil	9	23	63	10	53	5:1	+++
Wheatgerm oil	19	15	62	7	55	8:1	+

SFA saturated fatty acids
MUFA monounsaturated fatty acids
PUFA polyunsaturated fatty acids
Smoke points <150°C +; 150-200°C ++; >200°C +++[10]

The question of omega 3 and 6

Omega 6 fatty acids have been generally seen as pro-inflammatory and omega 3 as anti-inflammatory, so it has been understood that it is important to consume oils with as low a ratio of omega 6 to 3 as possible. To improve inflammation it has been suggested that we aim at a proportion of 3–4:1 omega 6:3 for all the oils and fats in the diet, but read on for different ideas.

However, although sesame oil is high in omega 6 fatty acids, it has been shown to be able to decrease high levels of inflammation and blood lipids, to reduce risk of atherosclerosis and to delay the onset of cardiovascular diseases.[11]

So how can this be squared with the understanding that omega 6 is bad and omega 3 is good?

It was thought that arachidonic acid, converted from linolenic acid, an omega 6 fatty acid, was promoting inflammation, but it is now recognised that arachidonic acid is not all bad, and actually has anti-inflammatory effects. Also very little linolenic acid is converted into arachidonic acid in the body.

Our current understanding seems to be that we need more omega 3 fats, but don't need to reduce omega 6 fats from healthy cold-pressed plant oils, which are all helpful at reducing cardiovascular disease.[12]

It is important to avoid rancid oils as they form lots of free radicals in the presence of oxygen, heat and light over time. This becomes pro-inflammatory, causes cellular damage and has been associated with diabetes, Alzheimer's disease and other inflammatory conditions. Saturated fats are much more stable, and less likely to go rancid than polyunsaturated fats.[13]

Non-cold pressed oils, which includes most cheap mass-produced oils, extract more oil from a given amount of plant material, but heat and sometimes solvents are used in the extraction. This creates a much less healthy oil, which is often rancid and contains carcinogenic free radicals. These are deodorised to prevent the smell of rancidity, so it is less easy to tell when they are old and rancid.

Cold pressed oils are also the more healthy option as they contain more antioxidant molecules and also more vitamin E, both of which are anti-inflammatory. So buy cold pressed, non-deodorised oils as fresh as possible, store them cool and dark and not for too long.

The other sources of good fats and oils include oily fish, especially wild oily fish such as sardines, mackerel and wild salmon, and grass-fed beef, lamb and game meats.

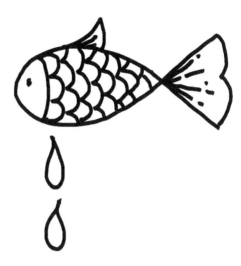

Diets

There are very many different diets, all of which have their benefits. It is important to try several different diets to see which is the best for the individual.

The **ketogenic diet** is often recommended as a good diet to reset the body especially where there is a dangerous level of inflammation. The ketogenic diet involves using fats as fuel rather than sugars or refined carbohydrates. It is high in fat and low in carbohydrates, and can be very helpful as a short-term reset for metabolic disease or cancer. However, it does include a lot of animal milk products, which are really not a good idea for most people, and it uses artificial sweeteners, which are definitely not a good idea as they keep the addictive nature of sweet tastes going.

The **Palaeo diet** aims to copy Palaeolithic man, the hunter gatherers who existed 10,000 years ago, before Neolithic man started farming. As far as we know, hunter gatherers foraged for fruit, vegetables, nuts, seeds and honey, and hunted for game meat, eggs and shellfish. It has been estimated that meat, eggs and fish made up about 35% of their diet with the remainder, 65%, being plant-based.[14]

There were no cultivated grains or dairy products in the Palaeolithic diet. Apparently the standard US diet in the twenty-first century includes about 10% non-grain plant-based foods, 24% grains, 9% dairy products, and 17% sugar and sweeteners. That's an enormously different diet, with the reduction in plant-based foods resulting in a much lower-fibre diet.

Human trials of Palaeo diets over as little as three weeks have all shown significant improvements in body weight, waist circumference and glucose tolerance.[15]

Dr Sarah Myhill has combined the Palaeo and ketogenic diets and removed most common allergens and addictive substances, and termed it the PK diet.[16]

Low glycaemic load diet. The low carbohydrate diets are not right for everyone, as some people need starches and whole grains in their diet. In this case a low glycaemic load diet may be helpful. This removes the high glycaemic load foods such as sugar, fructose corn syrup and refined grains from the diet, while keeping whole grains such as brown rice and oats.

Digestive recovery diet. This diet is suitable for anyone who has experienced long-term digestive inflammation and as a result has a sensitive and sore digestive tract. Often there is very poor nutrient absorption, so even though good foods are being eaten, the absorption of vitamins and minerals from the food is meagre – so as well as healing the digestive tract it is important that foods are easily digested.

It is important to eat little and often, and not overload the gut with a heavy meal. Eat something every three to four hours, but don't graze otherwise the stomach will be constantly trying to work – give it time off between meals and snacks. Try to eat the largest meal by midday, and never drink more than a small glass of fluid with a meal. Use spices such as black pepper, mustard, ginger, coriander or cumin with all food if possible to help digestion.

Bitter herbs can be taken to help with digestion, and usually before eating to prepare the gut for food. Other good ways to help prepare the gut for digestion include a teaspoonful of cider vinegar or lime juice in a little water, or chewing on a piece of crystallised ginger, or grated fresh ginger mixed with a little grated or desiccated coconut, salt and lime juice.

Bone broths made from grass-fed beef or lamb or organic chicken will help to heal the gut and provide good and easily absorbed nutrition. Put bones or a whole chicken or pieces (with meat, fat and connective tissue still on) into a big pan of water with some onions and carrots, and a little cider vinegar. Simmer slowly for 12 to 24 hours. Use a slow cooker or a low oven. Season and strain the stock and freeze in portions.

Inflammation

Use the bone broth as a drink or as a base for soups and casseroles. However, anyone with a sensitivity to histamine shouldn't take bone broths as they are very high in histamine.

Start the day with juice of half a lemon or lime in half a pint of hot or cool water. Add a little grated fresh ginger root if liked.

Breakfast
Suggestions include:

- either fresh or stewed fruit with soaked nuts and seeds
- or nut milk, i.e. warm oat, nut or rice milk plus ground nuts/seeds plus a teaspoonful of honey or maple syrup
- or porridge made with oats, millet or quinoa flakes and cooked in water with lots of whole or ground nuts and seeds added after cooking, with dried or fresh fruit if you like
- or eggs in any form – maybe with mushrooms or mashed leftover vegetables from the day before. Use fats and oils such as ghee, cold-pressed organic rapeseed oil, coconut butter or good beef dripping for cooking.
- or green smoothie (see below).

Snacks
These should be soaked nuts, seeds and fruit, sesame bars, homemade flapjacks or cakes with added nuts, seeds and dried fruit, rice or oat cakes or rye crackers or carrot/celery sticks with hummus or nut butter or any of the suggested breakfasts.

Lunch
This should be the main meal if possible. We recommend kicharee, which is made of one part mung dahl (or puy lentils, split peas or similar pulses) plus two parts brown rice simmered slowly with a lid on in six parts water or stock (bone broth could be used here). Season with salt, black pepper, ginger, cumin, coriander and fresh herbs as liked, and seasonal vegetables at the appropriate stage of cooking.

The rice and dahl will need 35 to 45 minutes' gentle simmer. Do not stir after all ingredients are added or the result will be mush! Add ghee, hemp seed oil, olive, avocado or similar oils to serve. Alternatively, stir-fry lots of vegetables plus fish, organic poultry, grass-fed beef or lamb, tofu or nuts with brown rice or quinoa; or any of the protein foods above with vegetables of any kind – roast, mashed or steamed.

Evening meals

These should be light. Try home-made soups, or salads with sprouted seeds – avocado would be good here, plus oils and spices as salad dressings. Use pulses, eggs, fish, nuts and seeds, tofu or organic chicken as your protein foods. A miso soup would also be good here with fine-chopped vegetables and tofu. If available, use fermented tofu.

Avoid all wheat, dairy, or processed foods and omit alcohol, tea or coffee, although one coffee or tea without animal milk is fine. Also avoid pork and oranges as they are too inflammatory, and keep sugar as low as possible. Try to eat organic foods as much as possible. Grass-fed red meat is fine in small portions only, and no more than once a day, preferably at lunchtime.

If the digestive tract is very sore, have a couple of days with just liquid foods, for example green smoothies, miso soup, chicken broth etc.

Take probiotics as capsules or unpasteurised fermented foods to replace bowel flora for a month or two – this will also help with digestion. Avoid fermented foods with histamine sensitivity as they are high in histamines.

After long-term digestive problems vitamin and mineral supplements may be needed short-term to repair any deficiencies. These will be best as liquid preparations as they will be more easily absorbed.

This is the best way to organise the meals, but lunch and evening meals can be swapped if it makes life easier. Drink plenty of fluids throughout the day, preferring water and herb teas, especially those with spices in such as ginger, fennel, cardamon, aniseed and celery seed.

The digestive recovery diet is useful for anyone who is just starting out on a gut-healing programme, and should be followed at least until symptoms improve. But it is also useful as a regular intermittent diet just to make sure the digestive system is healthy.

Food intolerance diets

Avoiding dairy products. Dairy products include anything made from the milk of any animal – cow, goat, sheep, buffalo. It doesn't include eggs. So that means no milk, yogurt, cheese, cream or ice cream, and it also means that it is important to check food labels for skimmed milk and whey powder, which are both put into many processed food products such as biscuits, milk chocolate, sweets, ready meals, soups etc.

Most people who are dairy intolerant can usually have butter in moderation. This is because butter is almost 100% dairy fat, and it is mostly either the proteins or the sugars in milk that cause the problem. For those who are hypersensitive to milk proteins it may be important to avoid butter and use ghee (clarified butter) instead.

Alternatives to milk are easy – use rice, oat, almond, hazelnut or coconut milks on cereals, in tea, for cooking – just the same way as ordinary milk. Coconut cream and oat cream can both be used as pouring creams or in cooking.

Homemade milks are easy. For oat milk, soak a cup of rolled oats in a litre of water for a short time, whizz in a blender, and strain through a fine sieve. Add a pinch of salt and a dash of hemp seed or olive oil, or a few drops of vanilla essence before blending if liked.

Use the same method for nuts, seeds or cooked brown rice. Nut or seed milks are better when they are soaked for a couple of hours.

Soya products are plentiful – ice cream, cheese, cream cheese, milk, yogurt and so on – but it is very important only to use these occasionally. Soya is allergenic, meaning that if soya products are eaten every day, several times a day, intolerance to soya will develop within a few months, and that will make life more difficult. So restrict soya products to no more than four or five times a week. Soya in excess will also suppress the thyroid gland.

There are plenty of excellent dairy-free products available in all shops now – ice creams, cheeses, yogurts, chocolates. But be wary of lactose-free milk products, which still contain milk protein so they are actually not useful for most dairy-intolerant people.

An alternative to grated cheese as a sprinkle on top of foods is to whizz any nuts or seeds in a mini-grinder with some salt, or grind them in a pestle and mortar. This sprinkle is very effective and nutritious. Try it on pasta dishes, but don't put it under the grill or in the oven to brown. Inactivated yeast flakes can also be sprinkled on food – soups, casseroles, salads – to supply a cheesy taste.

Calcium and magnesium can be obtained from many foods other than animal milks – especially good are nuts and seeds, sesame seeds in particular – and many of the alternative milks are also fortified with extra calcium. We don't need milk nutritionally once we are weaned –

remember it is food for babies, not adults, and contains many natural growth hormones that can, by themselves, cause further health problems.

Everybody has their own level of tolerance to dairy products. Some cannot cope with even the smallest amount, while others can tolerate it once a week, for example. It is important to determine one's own tolerance level by cutting out dairy completely for 8 to 12 weeks, see how that feels, and then reintroduce a small amount.

Just occasionally, in someone who eats a great deal of dairy products, removing it completely can cause withdrawal symptoms. This is not common but it does happen, and symptoms can actually be quite severe stomach pains. So in these people it is probably sensible to advise a slow withdrawal over a couple of weeks.

When the body is under stress – mental or physical – tolerance levels will be much lower than in a healthy body without stress. So if there is a viral infection, at exam time or house moving for example, dairy will need to be removed from the diet again. Some people also find that they can tolerate goat's or sheep's milk products more easily than cows – again, it's about finding the tolerance level of the individual.

Gluten-free diet. The gluten-containing grains are wheat, spelt, emmer, barley, rye and oats – some people can tolerate oats, others have to use gluten-free oats.

There are very many recipes available online – look up Palaeo recipes too.

The standard gluten-free flour mixes need extra fluids or oils as they can turn out rather dry and unappetizing, and some contain potato starch, which not everyone can take. My website http://www.christineherbert. co.uk has a number of my favourite gluten-free recipes.

Avoiding nightshade family foods. The common symptoms seen in nightshade intolerance are tissue inflexibility, which causes headaches, constipation, joint stiffness and pain, sometimes high blood pressure, and often eczema and sometimes neurological disorders.

The nightshade family of plants (Solanaceae) contain solanine, a glycoalkaloid that is more toxic to some people than others. Those who are sensitive to it can't eat potatoes, tomatoes, sweet and hot peppers, and aubergines. Tobacco is also in this family. Don't forget crisps, other potato snacks, gluten-free flour and many processed foods often contain potato.

It's fine to eat sweet potato, parsnip, swede, turnip and squash, all of which can be roasted, mashed or chipped just like potatoes.

Avoid nightshades completely for three months and then cautiously try a little – individual tolerance levels may permit occasional eating.

Unfortunately, unlike dairy and wheat, the symptoms of nightshade intolerance don't come and go as quickly. It can take weeks for them to appear and disappear.

Where recipes call for tomatoes there are a few useful substitutes that work well – for stews, Bolognese sauces and curries it is possible to use umeboshi plum paste, tamarind paste, pomegranate molasses, red wine or red wine vinegar – all have a tartness that works as a replacement for tomatoes.

Low-salicylate diet. Salicylates are present in all plants, so it is important to know which plants are high in salicylates and which are low, in order to be able to reduce the load on the body.

Salicylate sensitivity seems to be a transient problem for most, but not all, sufferers, so it is usually worth testing out one's sensitivity every now and again. Common issues with this food intolerance are digestive upsets, skin rashes and exacerbation of joint pains. For hypersensitive people it will be necessary to look at skin creams, shampoos and toothpastes – anything that touches the body – and this can be difficult as many do contain high-salicylate ingredients. Most salicylate-sensitive people are not this sensitive, fortunately.

Online there are many lists of salicylate-containing foods and their levels, but the reliability of these can vary enormously. There is probably no absolutely accurate list as the amount of salicylate in a plant will vary according to its growing conditions, climate, harvest time and so on.

The list provided here is one that I have found successful for most people I have looked after with salicylate sensitivity. There is also a list of high-salicylate herbs, but this is not exhaustive. Generally, removing the peel or skin from fruit and vegetables decreases the salicylate load.

Medicinal herbs that are high in salicylates include the following:

- *Arctostaphylos uva-ursi*
- *Arnica montana*

High salicylate fruits
Apricot
Black currant
Blackberry
Blueberry
Cherry
Cranberry
Goji berry
Gooseberry
Grape
Kiwi
Nectarine
Peach
Pineapple
Poemegranate
Raspberry
Red currant
Rhubarb
Strawberry

Medium salicylate fruits
Melon
Pear

Low salicylate fruits
Apple
Avocado
Banana
Date
Fig
Lemon
Lime
Mango
Orange
Papaya
Plum
Quince
Tamarind

High salicylate veg
Chilli
Courgette (zucchini)
Cucumber
Old potato skin
Pepper
Sweet potato
Tomato

Med. salicylate veg
Peeled cucumber
Peeled courgette
Skinned tomato
Tinned tomato

Low salicylate veg
Asparagus
Aubergine (eggplant)
Beetroot
Broccoli
Cabbage
Carrot
Cauliflower
Celery
Chard/spinach
Green beans
Lettuce/salad leaves
Muchrooms
Onion/shallot
Parsnip
Peas
Squash
Swede (rutabaga)
Turnip
Sweetcorn

Inflammation

High salicylate herbs & spices
Chamomile
Chilli
Cinnamon
Elderflower
Mint
Nutmeg
Oregano & Marjoram
Rose
Rosehip
Thyme
Turmeric

Med. salicylate herbs & spices
Cardamom
Clove
Coriander seed
Garlic

Low salicylate herbs & spices
Asafoetida
Basil
Black cumin (nigella)
Blackpepper
Caraway
Celery seed
Chervil
Coriander leaf
Cumin
Dill
Fennel
Fenugreek
Ginger
Horseradish
Lemon balm
Mustard
Parsley
Rosemary
Sage
Vanilla

Other high salicylate
All alcohol from grapes
Almonds
Aloe vera juice
Aspirin
Carob
Chocolate
Cocoa powder
Earl grey tea
Elderflower cordial
Liquorice
Peanuts
Wine

Other med. salicylate
Brazil nuts
Coconut
Coconut oil
Hemp seeds
Olives
Olive oil
Peanuts without skins

Other low salicylate
All grains
All pulses
Beer and cider
Black, green, and white tea
Cider vinegar
Coffee
Hazels, walnuts, pecans
Mayonnaise
Pine nuts, macadamia
Pumpkin seeds
Rapeseed oil
Sesame seeds
Soy sauce/tamari
Sugar
Sunflower seeds

- *Capsicum annum*
- *Cinnamomum*
- *Coleus forskohlii*
- *Corydalis* spp.
- *Curcuma longa*
- *Filipendula ulmaria*
- *Glycyrrhiza glabra, G. uralensis*
- *Hyssopus officinalis*
- *Iris versicolor*
- *Lycium chinense*
- *Lepidium meyenii*
- *Matricaria chamomilla*
- *Mentha* spp.
- *Mitchella repens*
- *Myristica fragrans*
- *Oreganum vulgare*
- *Phytolacca americana*
- *Prunus serotina*
- *Rehmannia* prep. (raw is low)
- *Rosa* spp. flower and hip
- *Salix* spp.
- *Sambucus nigra* flower and fruit
- *Schisandra chinensis*
- *Theobroma*
- *Thymus* spp.
- *Vaccinium myrtillus*
- *Vaccinium vitis idaea*
- *Vitex agnus castus*
- *Zanthoxylum* spp.

Oils that can be used for massage and skin care that are low in salicylates include shea butter, argan oil, jojoba oil and tamanu oil.

Be careful with toothpastes and mouthwashes containing mint of any kind.

Low-histamine diet. The best way to test for histamine intolerance is to follow a low-histamine diet and see if symptoms of inflammation disappear. These symptoms could be respiratory, digestive or skin reactions. They should disappear fairly quickly if a very low-histamine diet is followed, and reappear once they are reintroduced into the diet.

High-histamine foods include:

- alcohol, especially wine, cider and beer
- long-cooked or aged meat, especially when eaten as leftovers
- bone broths
- fermented foods, including meat, fish, vegetables, yogurt
- smoked meat and fish
- aged cheeses
- dried fruit
- citrus fruit, strawberries, avocadoes
- tomatoes, spinach, mushrooms
- nuts
- cinnamon
- chocolate
- also histamine-liberating foods, which include bananas, pineapple, shellfish and egg whites.

Other causes of histamine release in the body include stress, temperature extremes, high-energy exercise, massage, insect bites, and methyl forms of B vitamin supplements.

A low-histamine diet will consist initially of:

- fresh or freshly frozen meat or fish
- egg yolks
- gluten-free grains
- fruits: mango, pear, watermelon, apple, kiwi, melon, grapes
- vegetables: all except those listed above
- alternative milks, e.g. coconut, rice and hemp milks
- olive oil, coconut oil

before gradually reintroducing a few of the higher-histamine foods once symptoms have disappeared.[17,18]

Green smoothies
These are the ultimate health drink, are good for everyone, and supply plenty of vitamins, minerals and enzymes in a very assimilable way. They are better than taking vitamin pills and probably supply everything needed by the body except vitamin D3. They are also an excellent way to take the more palatable herbs.

All ingredients must be raw, as fresh as possible, and the green vegetables should be organic if available.

Into an ordinary blender put about 300ml of water. Add in the other ingredients a few at a time, blending until smooth.

Everything is optional except the lemon juice, something green and a little oil – make it with what you can find, and what you like. Use the list as a guide:

- any green leafy vegetable such as spinach, kale, rocket, lettuce
- wild herbs such as dandelion leaves, plantain leaves, cleavers, hawthorn buds and leaves,   stinging nettles, ground ivy
- cultivated herbs such as lemon balm, rosemary, mint, chives, parsley
- any sprouted seeds such as alfalfa
- cucumber
- pea shoots
- mange tout peas
- broccoli
- celery and celery leaf
- fennel bulb
- avocado
- chlorella 1–5 grams – start low and build up
- any commercial green superfood
- pinch of salt
- fresh juice of a half to one lemon, plus a little peel if it is organic/unwaxed
- garlic to taste
- any prescribed herbs can be added here, but are not essential
- a little olive or hemp seed oil and/or fish oils

Divide the smoothie into two servings. Drink one half straight away, and have the other half by lunch time. The second portion should be kept cool. Try to 'chew' as it is drunk, as downing it too quickly can cause bloating.

Fasting
Fasting has a lot of benefits for inflammatory disease. There are many ways of fasting, and again it is important to find the best way for the individual. The benefits of fasting include:

- Reduced inflammation via many processes. In the case of an acute inflammatory attack such as in autoimmune disease, the fastest way to reduce this is to do a two-day water fast. This has been recommended by physicians for several thousand years, and was suggested by Hippocrates.

- Improved cell regeneration. Autophagy, where dead and dysfunctional cells are removed and cell nutrients recycled, is increased.
- Improved gut healing: the digestive system is given a rest so it can heal.
- Production of ghrelin, the hunger hormone, is enhanced and as well as informing the body it needs to eat it also acts on the innate and adaptive immune systems to suppress inflammation and induce anti-inflammatory markers.[19]
- The effects of alterative and gut-healing herbs are greatly enhanced.
- Individuals undergoing short-term fasts of 1–2 days frequently report improvements in energy, mood, self-confidence and quality of life.[20]
- Calorie restriction elicits cell-protective responses in nearly all tissues and organs that extend lifespan. This is an evolutionary protective mechanism that ensures survival when faced with starvation.[21]
- Calorie restriction involves the downregulation of insulin, and reduction of inflammation.[22]

A review of studies of those fasting for the Muslim holy month of Ramadan where people fast for 12–20 hours a day for one month found several benefits as regards inflammation. Serum levels of several pro-inflammatory cytokines IL-6, IL-1beta, TNF-alpha, were significantly lower during Ramadan compared to pre- and post-Ramadan fasting. In cardiac patients there were significant benefits owing to reduced oxidative stress. There was a small reduction in weight, but this was accompanied by substantial decreases in indicators for metabolic syndrome – fasting blood sugar, systolic blood pressure, total triglycerides and waist circumference – as well as an increase in high-density cholesterol. It was also found that the immune system was better able to fight *Mycobacterium tuberculosis*, the causative pathogen for tuberculosis.[23]

Chapter summary:

- The elements of a general anti-inflammatory diet
- Food intolerances, and irritant foods
- Phytonutrients and where to find them
- Choosing oils and fats for an anti-inflammatory diet
- Diets for digestive recovery, and specific food intolerances
- Green smoothie
- The benefits of fasting

7
Other methods to reduce inflammation

Supplements
Although I am not a big fan of supplements, and would rather use natural foods where possible, sometimes vitamin and mineral supplements can be helpful, at least until an inflamed digestive system is healed and more able to absorb nutrients from food. Inflamed mucous membranes of the gastrointestinal tract don't function as well so there is less absorption of nutrients, and the actual process of inflammation uses up nutrients.

The nutrients that are most commonly deficient in many people are magnesium, vitamin D3, zinc, selenium and vitamin B6. The two supplements that most people need are magnesium and vitamin D3, and those with chronic inflammation may need more.

Vitamin A is vital for eye health, general growth and development, and protecting epithelium and mucus integrity in the body. It is necessary for immune system health and plays an important role in the inflammatory process.

It has been shown that supplementation will improve the functioning and health of the intestinal lining.[1]

Vitamin A promotes mucin secretion and improves the barrier function of all the mucous membranes including the mouth, lungs and intestines. Where there is vitamin A deficiency, the epithelial cell lining shrinks and hardens, and becomes unable to repel foreign pathogens and act as the first line of defence.[2]

Vitamin A supplementation has been found to reduce inflammation in several chronic inflammatory disease states, and its deficiency itself induces inflammation.[3]

B vitamins
A growing body of evidence supports the protective action of B vitamins in reducing inflammation in patients with inflammatory diseases and general populations.[4] B vitamins appear to be able to reduce inflammation as measured by reductions in both homocysteine and C-reactive protein. In particular, supplementation of vitamins B6, B9 (folate) and B12 have shown improvements in cardiovascular disease.[5]

Folate may reduce inflammation owing to its beneficial effects in scavenging free radicals and reactive oxygen species, and in lowering cholesterol and blood pressure that are associated with reducing inflammation.

One study concluded that a large dose of vitamin B6 supplementation (100mg/day) suppressed pro-inflammatory cytokines (specifically IL-6 and TNF-α) in patients with rheumatoid arthritis,[6] and that there seem to be higher demands for vitamin B6 when there is active inflammation.[7]

Vitamin C
Vitamin C is important to the proper functioning of the immune system as it supports many activities of both the innate and the adaptive systems. It supports epithelial barrier function against pathogens and protects against environmental oxidative stress. It accumulates in phagocytic cells and enhances their functions, as well as improving autophagy and apoptosis.
It also seems to have a role in both B and T-lymphocyte function. A deficiency of vitamin C results in lowered immunity and increased risk of infection. Immune system activation and inflammation for any cause uses excess amounts of vitamin C; this has been observed for many years, with scurvy being seen as a common after effect of infections in the past.

It is well recognised that supplementary vitamin C is important when there is infection, and also that requirements are higher when there is any toxic load or inflammatory process occurring in the body.

Vitamin C is not stored in the body so daily intake is important. It is a relatively common deficiency and is the fourth most common nutrient deficiency in the USA.[8]

As a strong antioxidant vitamin C is able to reduce inflammation by neutralising free radicals, which are pro-inflammatory. Vitamin C at 500mg twice daily was shown to decrease inflammatory markers C-reactive protein (CRP), IL-6, triglycerides and fasting blood glucose within just 8 weeks of its use in hypertensive and/or diabetic obese patients.[9]

It is well established that vitamin C inhibits oxidation of LDL-protein, and current research suggests that vitamin C deficiency is associated with a higher risk of mortality from cardiovascular disease and that vitamin C may improve endothelial function and lipid profiles in some groups, especially those with low plasma vitamin C levels.[10]

Vitamin C is important in skin health, both as an antioxidant and as a vital factor in collagen synthesis and hence skin repair. It has been found to be deficient in those with inflammatory skin diseases and its supplementation shown to be helpful.[11]

When needed for inflammation vitamin C can be taken to bowel tolerance, that is, until the dose causes diarrhoea, and then reduced enough so that no ill effect is felt. This might be as high as 8–15g per day. It is best taken in separate doses throughout the day to maintain high blood levels. A standard dose for maintenance is 1–2g daily.

Vitamin D3
Vitamin D 3 is another vital vitamin for the immune system. It acts as an immunomodulator, specifically with strong anti-inflammatory effects. Its deficiency is very prevalent, especially in regions where people don't get sun exposure on the skin for many months of the year, as this is the best way to get good amounts of vitamin D3.

A deficiency is strongly associated with all the inflammatory diseases, and it has become increasingly common for the medical profession to suggest that everyone should take a supplement through the winter.[12]

Vitamin D3 levels are measured as serum concentration of 25(OH)D; adequate levels are said to be at least 50nmol/litre (20ng/ml). This may be an underestimate and more may well be better. More than 75% of people with a variety of cancers have low levels of vitamin D, and the lowest levels are associated with the more advanced cancers.[13]

The deficiency has been found to be more prevalent in those with diabetes and obesity, and it is also associated with vulnerability to infection, including coronavirus and pneumonia, and also an increase in inflammatory cytokines, which tends to increase severity of infection.

Vitamin D3 deficiency is associated with an increase in thrombotic episodes, which are also seen in COVID-19.[14] Intake of 2,000iu vitamin D3 daily has been shown to improve intestinal permeability and to reduce CRP plasma levels in patients with inflammatory bowel disease.[15]

There is some evidence that vitamin D deficiency is associated with an increased risk for vascular diseases and it also increases general mortality.[16]

Vitamin D is formed in skin after exposure to ultraviolet-B radiation (UVB), which enters the bloodstream and undergoes hydroxylation in the liver to 25-hydroxyvitamin D (25(OH)D). This is the major circulating form of vitamin D and is used as a measure of vitamin D status. This is further hydroxylated in the kidney to 1,25-dihydroxyvitamin D (1,25(OH)2D), which is the active form. However, a factor 15 sunscreen can reduce D3 production in the body by 99%.[17]

Ten minutes of midday sun on the skin (forearms and lower legs exposed) between March and September will provide enough vitamin D3 for the year, assuming pale skin and adequate levels of D3 at the start. Those with darker skins need up to 45 minutes a day.[18]

Supplementation is probably a good idea, especially in the winter months, and especially when there is increased demand with chronic inflammation. Assuming adequate levels initially (this really needs a blood test to determine), then a maintenance dose for those with inflammatory disorders should be between 2,000 and 6,000iu daily.[19]

Magnesium status is also important as suboptimal levels of magnesium will reduce activation of D3 in the body.

Vitamin E
Vitamin E is another powerful antioxidant with beneficial actions on inflammation. Vitamin E is actually a group of fat-soluble chemicals that include tocopherols and tocotrienols, most of which are antioxidants. It is the most abundant fat-soluble antioxidant present in body tissues, and it has a beneficial effect on the prevention and management of chronic diseases including stroke, hypertension, diabetes and fatty liver disease.

Vitamin E has been shown to inhibit inflammatory cytokine expression, and a link between vitamin E intake and blood levels of cytokines is favourable.[20]

Vitamin E is able to inhibit COX-2, an enzyme involved in inflammatory reactions. Studies on inflammation and osteoporosis have found that vitamin E is able to neutralise free radicals involved in the production of bone-resorbing cytokines, resulting in reduced bone destruction. In patients with coronary artery disease vitamin E was shown to reduce inflammation as they exhibited a decrease in CRP and tumour necrosis factor-alpha (TNF-alpha). It is also believed to exert anti-inflammatory and anti-carcinogenic activity in the intestines, especially the colon.[21]

Magnesium
Magnesium is involved in hundreds of biochemical reactions in the body and is found in all body tissues, with 60% of total magnesium occurring in the bones. Every cell in the body has a requirement for magnesium. Func-

tions include creating and repairing RNA and DNA, protein formation, muscle function and nervous system regulation.

Magnesium is very commonly deficient in diets, and supplementation can be very helpful for many people. A 2005 survey in the USA found that about 60% of adults did not obtain the estimated average requirement of magnesium daily.[22] As more than 99% of total body magnesium is found in tissue cells and very little in blood, most cases of magnesium deficiency are undiagnosed.

If the body is deficient in magnesium then many body functions are inefficient, and this includes muscle function. Muscles don't relax properly when they are deficient in magnesium, and if muscles can't relax then the body can't relax into sleep.

Magnesium deficiency is extremely common. The official journal of the British Cardiovascular Society published a paper which concluded that:

"Subclinical magnesium deficiency is a common and under-recognised problem throughout the world. Importantly, subclinical magnesium deficiency does not manifest as clinically apparent symptoms and thus is not easily recognised by the clinician. Despite this fact, subclinical magnesium deficiency likely leads to hypertension, arrhythmias, arterial calcifications, atherosclerosis, heart failure and an increased risk for thrombosis."[23]

Symptoms suggesting magnesium deficiency include restless legs, restless sleep, premenstrual syndrome, muscle aches and pains, and tension headaches. Many of these can be helped by simply taking 500–1,000mg magnesium citrate daily, or soaking in an Epsom salts bath. Sluggish bowels or constipation will also be improved.

Low mood and depression can improve with magnesium supplementation.[24]

Magnesium deficiency itself is pro-inflammatory. It has been shown to activate phagocytic cells, release inflammatory cytokines and produce excess free radicals. The mechanism by which this happens may include the role of magnesium as a calcium channel blocker. A deficiency increases cellular calcium, and also sodium, which signals the cells to activate the inflammatory response.

Magnesium deficiency becomes a risk factor for many chronic inflammatory conditions, including cardiovascular disease, diabetes and hypertension. One study of non-diabetic, non-hypertensive but obese people found raised TNF-alpha inflammatory marker and reduced serum magnesium levels.[25]

A craving for dark chocolate can often be an indication of magnesium deficiency as dark chocolate is very high in magnesium. Other good sources are pumpkin seeds, dark green leafy vegetables, nuts and oily fish.

Those taking a calcium supplement might well find they are precipitating a magnesium deficiency as excess calcium reduces the availability of magnesium in the body.

A meta-analysis of eight randomised and controlled trials showed that magnesium supplementation of between 320 and 500mg daily significantly decreased CRP levels.[26] It is therefore always going to be useful to supplement with magnesium with any chronic inflammatory condition.

Zinc

Zinc is an essential micronutrient that acts as an antioxidant, plays an important role in both innate and adaptive immunity, and acts as an anti-inflammatory agent. The main cause of deficiency worldwide is malnutrition, but even in developed countries it has been estimated that nearly 30% of elderly people are deficient in zinc.[27]

Zinc can influence the production and signalling of many inflammatory cytokines, and plasma levels can be seen to drop rapidly when there is acute infection, stress or trauma, as zinc is moved into cells in order to support the body. Every immunological event is influenced by zinc.

As there are no storage facilities for zinc in the body, it needs to be taken daily to maintain good levels. Foods with the highest zinc concentration include red meat, some shellfish, legumes and wholegrains. However, zinc from animal sources is more bioavailable to the body.

Supplementation is also possible, and probably advisable when there is increased demand, such as infection or inflammation, and the most bioavailable supplements are those bound to amino acids such as zinc aspartate, cysteine or histidine. Zinc oxide is very poorly bioavailable.[28]

Selenium

Dietary selenium plays an important role in inflammation and immunity. Adequate levels both initiate immunity and also regulate excessive immunity and chronic inflammation.

Dietary selenium is found in grains, vegetables, seafood, meat, dairy products and nuts, with the richest sources being brazil nuts, organ meats and seafood.

Inadequate selenium results in increased oxidative stress in immune cells at all stages of their function.[29] In a variety of diseases, selenium deficiency is likely to sustain inflammation and promote disease: cardiovascular disease, atherosclerosis, stroke, chronic pancreatitis, autoimmune disease, metabolic disease and chronic renal disease.

As chronic inflammation is believed to deplete selenium stores in the body, supplementation may be helpful where there is prolonged inflammation as selenium is the trace element most affected by it. This may also be useful in bacterial or viral infection.[30]

Fish oils
Omega 3 fatty acids as found in oily fish and fish oils are able to decrease the production of inflammatory eicosanoids, cytokines and reactive oxygen species. Omega 3 fatty acids are also used by the body to make specialised pro-resolving mediators (SPM). These are produced via the enzymatic conversion of essential fatty acids, including the omega 3 fatty acids docosahexaenoic acid and n-3 docosapentaenoic acid. These mediators exert protective actions reducing vascular and systemic inflammation.[31]

The benefits of fish oil supplementation have been controversial, with varying results of many studies. However, a review of studies of fish oil effect on hypertension concludes that it does have a significant lowering effect at a dose of 2g daily.[32] Another study showed that omega 3 fatty acids improved endogenous fibrinolysis and endothelial function, which may represent important mechanisms through which omega 3 fatty acids confer potential cardiovascular benefits.[33]

Many clinical trials of fish oil supplements have been carried out over the last thirty years on inflammatory diseases. Best outcomes have been seen in rheumatoid arthritis, osteoarthritis, systemic lupus erythematosus and lupus nephritis.[34]

Meditation practices
Meditation practices include meditation, yoga, Qigong, Tai Chi and other similar practices. It has long been known within groups that use these practices that they have a positive influence on chronic inflammatory disease. A review of fifteen studies of yoga and inflammation concluded that yoga will reduce inflammation across a multitude of chronic conditions.[35]

There is evidence that mind–body practice calms the activity of genes associated with inflammation, which can reverse inflammatory damage caused by stress. Another study, which analysed 18 trials covering over 800 participants, found that genes related to inflammation became less active. In particular there was an association with a downregulation of the nuclear factor kappa B pathway, which is the opposite of the effects of chronic stress on gene expression. This results in a reduced risk of chronic inflammatory disease.[36]

Another study compared the effects of mindfulness meditation with a relaxation retreat that had no mindfulness meditation element. This study looked at brain scans and interleukin-2 measurements in order to evaluate effects on inflammation, finding that mindfulness meditation reduced IL-2 inflammatory markers much more than relaxation. Brain scans showed improvements in the brain's functional connectivity, that is, the brain areas that typically work in opposition – mind-wandering and internal reflection as opposed to attention, planning and decision-making, were now working more in harmony. This harmony was better able to help the brain cope with stress, which was the reason for reduced inflammatory markers.[37]

A study that examined a group of people with inflammatory bowel disease (IBD) found that breathing exercises and Qigong had a beneficial result on IBD. The group had weekly sessions and practised for 20 minutes a day at home.

After just 6 weeks of this they had significantly improved anxiety, stress, depression and physical symptoms, and after 26 weeks C-reactive protein was significantly reduced, showing a reduction in inflammation. The control group, who had the same amount of sessions provided to the test group, but with sessions that were purely educational, teaching about IBD and stress, had no such improvements.[38]

Exercise
It is clear that a lack of physical activity contributes to chronic inflammatory disease, and many studies have shown that regular cardiovascular exercise can reduce markers of inflammation. This needs to be gradually introduced as acute unaccustomed exercise can actually cause inflammation.

Of all the randomised trials, those that showed a positive result where inflammation is reduced with exercise are those where the exercise had been continued for six months or more.

There are several possible mechanisms for this reduction. Regular exercise reduces fat mass and adipose tissue inflammation, which contributes to systemic inflammation; exercise increases muscle production of IL-6, which is known to reduce TNF-alpha production and increase anti-inflammatory cytokines; and exercise increases vagal tone, which can also reduce inflammation.[39,40]

Medication

Nonsteroidal anti-inflammatory drugs (NSAIDs) are efficacious analgesics, and antipyretics and are among the most frequently used drugs worldwide. They include aspirin and ibuprofen as well as much stronger prescription-only drugs such as diclofenac, indomethacin and COX-2 inhibitors such as celebrex and vioxx.

Vioxx and celebrex were hailed as the new wonder drugs because they had fewer side effects on the digestive system, and by 2004 at least 600,000 people were prescribed them in the UK. Unfortunately, research showed that they doubled their risk of heart attack, so vioxx has now been withdrawn and celebrex is not commonly prescribed any more.

Side effects of NSAIDS are commonly gut-related and include gastro-intestinal irritation and inflammation, caused by increasing gut permeability,[41] which increases the inflammatory process in the body.[42]

NSAIDs enteropathy arises from the enterohepatic recycling of drugs, resulting in a prolonged and repeated exposure of the intestinal mucosa to the compound and its metabolites. The impairment of the intestinal barrier represents the initial damage of NSAIDs enteropathy that leads to the translocation of bacteria and toxic substances of intestinal origin in the portal circulation, promoting an endotoxaemia.

This condition, mostly in patients with risk factors for nonalcoholic fatty liver disease, such as obesity and metabolic syndrome, might lead to liver inflammatory response that could promote the development of nonalcoholic steatohepatitis.[43]

This all increases the risk of cardiovascular disease, specifically stroke, heart attack or high blood pressure,[44] even when taken relatively short term.[45] Studies have also shown long-term use of NSAIDS results in nephrotoxicity and chronic kidney disease.[46]

NSAIDS may help with pain but they do nothing to resolve the underlying problem.

Metformin is commonly used in the treatment of type 2 diabetic patients with dyslipidemia and low-grade inflammation. The anti-inflammatory activity of metformin is evident by reductions in circulating TNF-alpha, IL-1beta, CRP and fibrinogen in these patients.[47]

Statins are used to reduce bio mediators of inflammation, but they can cause inflammation, particularly muscle inflammation as a relatively common side effect in some people, which can occasionally be serious.

The other prescribed drugs for inflammation are **corticosteroids**, hormonal anti-inflammatory agents. Examples include prednisone and cortisone. These are very strong medications with potentially severe side effects and tend only to be used as a last resort when it is critical to reduce inflammation as quickly as possible. Ideally they are used short-term, but once on them it can be difficult to come off them. They should be tapered off very slowly and gradually with the guidance of the prescribing medic.

Chapter summary:

- Vitamin and mineral function and relationship with inflammation
- The effects of meditation and exercise on inflammation.
- A brief description of medications used to reduce inflammation.

8
Using herbs to reduce inflammation

As we said in the first chapter, chronic inflammation has similar features to acute inflammation – vasodilation, increased blood flow and increased capillary permeability – creating pain, redness, swelling, heat and loss of or reduced function. But if it continues too long, owing to continued injury or because the process is suppressed, it can start to stagnate as the increased permeability resulting from tissue damage stops the proper flow of fluids. This results in stagnation.

Stagnation causes the build-up of byproducts of inflammation, which become toxic in excess. Stagnation causes more pain and eventually cold rather than heat as fluid movement is slowed down. The body's defence system can't clear this up now, and degenerative disease takes hold. This can be localised initially but it will become systemic eventually. Then tissue gets destroyed by inflammation, and stops functioning as well as it should.

The gut lining is very fast-dividing and hence is in the front line when things go wrong, but it is equally able to repair quickly when things improve. When cells behave abnormally there is more chance that they will become cancerous. The immune system is less strong so it can't weed out abnormal cells or fight infections. Cold and stagnation become the main characteristics of chronic inflammation.

So we need to stimulate, activate and heal the tissue where the problem is – using stimulant, alterative and tonic herbs that will increase cellular activity and encourage elimination of the impurities that are causing irritation and inflammation.

Stimulant herbs
These herbs stimulate the vital force to action; they can also be said to be herbs whose actions quicken and enliven the physiological activity of the body. They can be classed as stimulant laxatives, circulatory stimulants, bitter stimulants and so on.

It is easy to overstimulate especially if someone is debilitated, so it is always advisable to go cautiously and gradually with treatment. Some people will need drop doses of these herbs, with a slowly increasing dose.

Stimulant herbs often act on particular organs or body systems, and others act on several areas of the body; some are cooling and some warming, so they can be chosen to suit the individual constitution. Some examples follow:

Cardiovascular stimulants

- Prickly ash *Zanthoxylum americanum* (warming)
- Rosemary *Salvia rosmarinus* (warming)
- Yarrow *Achillea millefolium* (cooling)
- Cayenne *Capsicum annuum* (warming)
- Ginger *Zingiber officinale* (warming)

Respiratory stimulants

- Angelica *Angelica archangelica* (warming)
- Pleurisy root *Asclepias tuberosa* (cooling)
- Garlic *Allium sativum* (warming)
- Horseradish *Armoracia rusticana* (warming)
- Ground ivy *Glechoma hederacea* (cooling)
- Peppermint *Mentha piperita* (warming)
- White horehound *Marrubium vulgare* (cooling)
- Yarrow *Achillea millefolium* (cooling)

Lymphatic stimulants

- Iris *Iris versicolor* (cooling)
- Poke root *Phytolacca decandra* (cooling)
- Echinacea *Echinacea purpurea, E. angustifolia* (cooling)
- Yellow dock *Rumex crispus* (cooling)

Digestive stimulants (including the bitter stimulant herbs)

- Angelica *Angelica archangelica* (warming)
- Blessed thistle *Carbenia benedicta* (cooling)
- Goldenseal *Hydrastis canadensis* (cooling)
- Barberry *Berberis vulgaris* (cooling)
- Senna *Senna* sp. (cooling)
- Yellow dock *Rumex crispus* (cooling_
- Dandelion *Taraxacum officinale* root (cooling)

Digestive aromatic stimulants

- Celery seed *Apium graveolens* (warming)
- Cinnamon *Cinnamomum* spp. (warming)

- Garlic *Allium sativum* (warming)
- Peppermint *Mentha piperita* (warming)
- Rosemary *Salvia rosmarinus* (warming)
- Black pepper *Piper nigrum* (warming)

Urinary stimulants

- Gravel root *Eupatorium purpureum* (cooling)
- Buchu *Barosma betulina* (warming)
- Yarrow *Achillea millefolium* (cooling)

Musculoskeletal stimulants

- Ginger *Zingiber officinale* (warming)
- Cayenne *Capsicum annuum* (warming)

Nervous system stimulants

- Coffee *Coffea arabica* (warming)
- Tea *Camellia sinensis* (warming)

Alterative herbs
These increase elimination of waste products from the body by making the process more effective.

Alteratives may need to be very gently applied as those who are fragile may not be able to cope with their strength; they are contraindicated in someone who has a very dry constitution.

Alterative herbs are covered in detail at the end of chapter 4.

Tonic herbs
Some tonic herbs are adaptogens, but many are not. Tonics tend to act on one or two body systems, but adaptogens work more generally in the body.

Tonics alleviate conditions of weakness in the body. A tonic herb is able to restore, tone and invigorate a body system. Most tonic herbs are like foods – indeed some of them are foods – they are safe, easily digestible and assimilable. They balance the organ system or the whole body, and restore homeostasis. Most (maybe all) are also inflammation-mediating.

Physiomedicalist herbalists call them trophorestoratives because they nourish and strengthen a body system. In traditional Chinese medicine (TCM) tonic herbs supplement deficiencies and enhance energy and well-being, and are contraindicated in damp conditions.

Tonic herbs include:

Immune system tonics

- Astragalus root *Astragalus membranaceus*
- Elecampane root *Inula helenium*
- Reishi *Ganoderma lucidum*

Bitter digestive system tonics

- Angelica *Angelica archangelica*
- Agrimony *Agrimonia eupatoria*
- Barberry *Berberis vulgaris*
- Artichoke *Cynara scolymus*
- Gentian *Gentiana lutea*
- Goldenseal *Hydrastis canadensis*

Respiratory tonics

- Goldenrod *Solidago virgaurea*
- Elecampane root *Inula helenium*
- Liquorice root *Glycyrrhiza glabra*
- Eyebright *Euphrasia officinalis* (tonic to the eyes and upper respiratory mucous membranes)
- Ground ivy *Glechoma hederacea*

Cardiac tonics
These can vitalise heart blood and improve circulation

- Ginkgo *Ginkgo biloba*
- Hawthorn berry *Crataegus* spp.
- Linden flower *Tilia europaea*
- Garlic *Allium sativum*
- Yarrow *Achillea millefolium*
- Daisy *Bellis perennis*

Inflammation

Urinary system tonics

- Fennel seed *Foeniculum vulgare*
- Burdock root *Arctium lappa*
- Heartsease *Viola tricolor*
- Gravel root *Eupatorium purpureum*
- Asparagus root *Asparagus racemosus*
- Yarrow *Achillea millefolium*
- Stinging nettle *Urtica dioica*

Reproductive system tonics

- Raspberry leaf *Rubus idaeus*
- Rose *Rosa* spp.
- Saw palmetto *Serenoa repens*
- Damiana leaf *Turnera aphrodisiaca*

Adaptogens
This class of herbs can be considered tonics as well as adaptogens. They do all that tonics do, and more. Adaptogenic herbs:

- Are non-toxic.
- Are often amphoteric, that is, they normalise or balance an organ or system when it has become unbalanced, whether overactive or under-active.
- Have antioxidant activity.
- Produce a non-specific defence response to stress.
- Can normalise physiological function and support homeostasis.
- Can regulate the two master control systems in the body, namely the hypothalamic–pituitary–adrenal (HPA) axis, and the sympathoadrenal system (SAS), that is, they help regulate the endocrine, nervous, immune, digestive and cardiovascular systems.

The current accepted definition is that adaptogens are 'a class of metabolic regulators that increase the ability of an organism to adapt to environmental factors and to avoid damage from such factors'.[1]

Adaptogens might be more suitable starting herbs for someone elderly, fragile or just very dry, instead of alteratives. Adaptogenic herbs include:

- Ashwagandha *Withania somnifera*
- Ginseng *Panax ginseng*
- Eleuthero *Eleutherococcus senticosus*

- Rose root *Rhodiola rosea*
- Reishi mushroom *Ganoderma lucidum*
- Holy basil *Ocimum sanctum* *
- Shatavari *Asparagus racemosus* *
- Astragalus *Astragalus membranaceus* *
- Gotu cola *Centella asiatica* *
- Nettle seed *Urtica dioica* sem *
- Rosemary *Salvia rosmarinus* *
- Burdock *Arctium lappa* rad & sem *

* not all herbalists agree that these are adaptogens, but they certainly come close and can be used in the same way as the classic adaptogens.

Inflammation-mediating herbs

Inflammation-mediating herbs work in very many different ways. They don't target a particular enzyme or action, but have many different constituents that act on a variety of targets. This results in a more gentle, safer action, admittedly not as strong as medication, but with far fewer side effects, and generally with a long-term healing approach rather than the temporary sticking plaster of medications.

An example is a study where knee osteoarthritis was treated for two months with either boswellia *Boswellia serrata* or valdecoxib (a NSAID). At the end of the two months both treatments were withdrawn; the positive effects of boswellia lasted an extra month, but the positive effects of valdecoxib ceased immediately.[2]

Many herbs have the ability to inhibit COX-2, without the side effects of the single-element COX-2 inhibitors. They include the berberine-containing herbs, barberry *Berberis vulgaris*, goldenseal *Hydrastis canadensis* and oregon grape *Mahonia aquifolium*. Other herbs able to inhibit COX-2 are holy basil *Ocimum sanctum*, turmeric *Curcuma longa*, Baikal skullcap *Scutellaria baicalensis*, Japanese knotweed *Polygonum cuspidatum*, rosemary *Salvia rosmarinus*, ginger *Zingiber officinale*, oregano *Origanum vulgare*, feverfew *Tanacetum parthenium*, and hops *Humulus lupulus*.[3]

A literature review of the effects of plant extracts on cytokine modulation showed the following list of medicinal plants had all been found to modulate at least one cytokine, and most modulated several:

- Astragalus *Astragalus membranaceus*
- Garlic *Allium sativum*
- Turkey tail fungus *Trametes versicolor*

- Turmeric *Curcuma longa*
- Echinacea *Echinacea purpurea*
- Maitake fungus *Grifola frondosa*
- Devil's claw *Harpagophytum procumbens*
- Korean ginseng *Panax ginseng*
- Milk thistle *Silybum marianum*
- Sarsaparilla *Smilax glabra*
- Guduchi *Tinospora cordifolia*
- Cat's claw *Uncaria tomentosa*
- Ashwaghanda *Withania somnifera* [4]

It appears that most, maybe all herbs, have a positive influence on inflammation in one way or another. See the appendix for a chart of the major inflammation-mediating herbs and their areas of action.

Mucilaginous herbs
Mucilage is a complex polysaccharide that has a demulcent or soothing effect on mucous membranes. Mucilage is found in many plants, and when mixed with water it becomes slimy, thick and coating.

The mucous membranes of the digestive and urinary tracts can be treated with these herbs by using them as teas or powders; they are very soothing to inflamed or irritated membranes in, for example, cystitis or irritable bowel syndrome.

Mucilaginous herbs include:

- Marshmallow *Althaea officinalis*
- Linseed *Linum usitatissimum*
- Plantain *Plantago lanceolate, P. major*
- Slippery elm *Ulmus fulva*

Methods of taking the herbs
Fresh herbs can simply be eaten in a salad, such as dandelion, centella or hawthorn leaves, or can be added to a green smoothie (see chapter 6 for a green smoothie recipe).

Herb teas or **infusions.** Just pour a cup of boiling water onto a teaspoon of dried herbs or a small handful of fresh herbs, and leave to sit until cool enough to drink. This can be drunk hot or cold. This can be of single herbs, such as chamomile, mint or lemon balm, or it can be of herbal combinations. If a sweet taste is desired then add in a little liquorice root – not too much or too often if there is high blood pressure.

Generally infusions are made with soft aerial parts of plants such as leaves and flowers. Sometimes an infusion can be made with cold water overnight – mucilaginous herbs such as marshmallow do well with a cold infusion.

Herbal decoctions are where harder plant materials such as seeds, barks and roots are simmered gently for anything from five minutes to half an hour. This might be the technique used for burdock or dandelion root. Again a little liquorice can be added if desired. But spices are also nice here, such as cardamom or cinnamon.

All these herbs can also be given as liquid extracts in the form of **tinctures** (these contain alcohol) or **glycerates** (these contain less or no alcohol). Tinctures are made by soaking the chopped herb in vodka or similar spirits for a couple of weeks in a glass jar. Use as little vodka as possible while making sure that the herb is covered, pressing it down well. Mix it regularly and after two to four weeks put it through a fine sieve or jelly bag, squeezing the liquid out as much as possible. This liquid tincture will keep for several years in a dark, cool place. It doesn't need refrigerating.

A glycerate is made in exactly the same way but instead of vodka use 70–80% vegetable glycerine plus 20–30% vodka, greatly reducing the amount of alcohol. It is possible to replace the vodka in a glycerate with water or a herb tea, but the glycerate is then prone to fermentation unless kept in the fridge.

Liquid herbal extracts can also be made in **cider vinegar** in the same way, but will need refrigeration to keep it for longer than a few months.

Herb powders can be taken mixed into any liquid, and are particularly effective taken in a green smoothie. See the recipe for green smoothie in chapter 6. Or they can be put into empty capsules.

Sweets can be made with any herb powders as follows:

- Put any dried fruit into a food processor and process until it becomes a solid mass.
- Add in any nuts or seeds, or nut or seed butter and process again.
- Add any other flavourings such as cocoa powder, rose or orange flower water or desiccated coconut. These quantities don't need measuring, but it is important to have a measured amount of your herb powders. Teaspoonfuls will do, and the measured amount could be a week's supply of herb powders at the correct dose. So mix that into

Inflammation

the food processor too.

- Then make balls with fingers of the mixture, and if two balls a day make the correct dose, for one week make 14 balls. These will keep in the fridge for the week.

A **chest balm** or **ointment** can be as simple as adding 10% by weight of beeswax to any base oil (such as olive oil), or any infused oil (such as calendula in olive oil) and heat gently until the beeswax is dissolved. Then add 2–3% of essential oil(s). Pour into jars and allow to set. Or mix the essential oils into any cream or ointment.

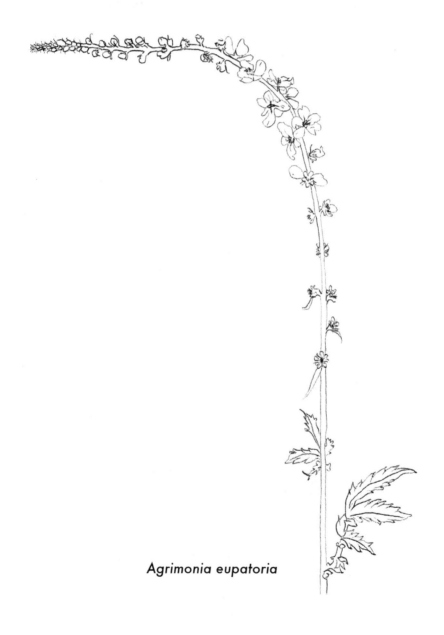

Agrimonia eupatoria

Inflammation

9
Materia medica

In the herb descriptions that follow I have mostly included those actions and properties that are relevant to chronic inflammation, so the descriptions are not always comprehensive and complete.

Dosage is very variable for all herbs. Some people do well with drop doses, and others need teaspoonfuls several times a day. Unless dosage is critical for a herb there are no guides given in this section, and if in doubt start low and slowly increase to see what works.

Guidance is given here as to which preparation is the best for each herb. At the end of this section is a glossary of terms.

Achillea millefolium **yarrow, aerial par**ts
Yarrow is a herb that has very many uses, but they mostly can be distilled to the fact that it improves blood circulation. It does this by acting as a vascular decongestant, peripheral vasodilator, antispasmodic and inflammation mediator.

It is used for many vascular issues including hypertension.[1] It is effective both to stop excessive bleeding and also to move any areas of blood stagnation or pooling. This quality can be used to help ease pain and aid healing in congested areas where there is bruising or varicosity, or painful periods, toothache, sinus congestion or headaches.

Yarrow acts as an inflammation-mediating herb systemically, and is often included in formulae to reduce inflammation and improve function in the lungs, liver and digestive system. As yarrow is also bitter this supports its function in the liver and digestive system.It can be taken as a tea or tincture, and is best made with fresh herb in flower.

Agrimonia eupatoria **agrimony, aerial parts**
Agrimony is a cooling, astringent and bitter herb, which acts as a tonic to digestion, the urinary system and the liver. It contains inflammation-mediating flavonoids and is a strong antioxidant; agrimony has been shown to improve markers of lipid metabolism, oxidative status and inflammation from as little as one month's consumption of agrimony tea.[2]

Agrimony is most useful where there is tension of any kind, for example where pain is preventing relaxation. American herbalist Matthew Wood considers agrimony to be specific where someone is holding their breath to reduce pain,[3] and he says agrimony will help them to breathe through the pain. This might be pain of breathing such as in inflammatory lung conditions, kidney or bladder pain, or digestive system pain. As a bitter astringent tonic, agrimony will help any inflammatory bowel condition where there is diarrhoea, or where there is evidence of underfunctioning liver and gallbladder with loose, yellow, floating stools.

Agrimony can be taken as tea, tincture or flower remedy, and is best harvested when it is in flower.

Agropyron repens **couch grass root**
Couch grass root is a very useful herb as a tea for bladder or prostate irritation, inflammation and pain. It has a demulcent and diuretic action. It is often mixed with other herbs such as corn silk *Zea mays* or marshmallow leaf *Althaea officinalis*.

When the bladder is irritated or painful it is good to drink as much of these herbs as tea as possible, even up to ten to twenty cups a day for a few days.

Allium sativum **garlic**
Garlic is a respiratory, immune and circulatory stimulant as well as being an excellent antimicrobial agent. It can also scavenge free radicals and act as an antioxidant.

There have been numerous research articles published citing garlic's activity as an anticancer agent. Most of its biological effects are attributed to organosulfur compounds including diallyl sulfide (DAS), diallyl disulfide (DADS), δ-glutamyl-S-allyl-L-cysteines, S allylmercaptocysteine (SAMC) and S-allyl-L-cysteine sulfoxides.[4]

Garlic is invaluable in respiratory infection where it acts as an expectorant as well as an antimicrobial. As it is very heating it should not be used for too long in hot conditions.

Aloe vera **aloe**
Aloe vera gel is the mucilaginous gel found inside the leaves of the aloe plant. This is demulcent to inflamed tissues, cooling and reducing inflammation to relieve the pain of irritation, bites and stings. It can be used topically or internally.

Althaea officinalis **marshmallow leaf and root**
This is a demulcent herb, very soothing and healing to mucous mem-

branes throughout the body. It is often used as a hot or cold infusion, or as a powder to help conditions involving inflammation or irritation of the bladder or digestive system. It is excellent mixed with lime flower *Tilia europaea* as a tea to help insomnia.

Andrographis paniculata **andrographis**
Andrographis is called the king of bitters, and is an important medicinal plant in many countries. It is very bitter and cooling, and has been used traditionally for fevers, malaria, dysentery and for venomous bites and stings. Research has suggested it is anticancer, antimicrobial (including HIV and hepatitis), inflammation-mediating, immune-stimulating, hypoglycaemic, antioxidant and hepatoprotective.[5]

It is most commonly used to combat infection, particularly of the lungs, liver and digestive tract, where it is antimicrobial and inflammation-mediating. Andrographis is a herb to use short-term in most cases, as it can cause digestive irritation when used longer-term.

As it is so bitter it is best taken as powder in capsules or as tincture. It is contraindicated in pregnancy or when breastfeeding.

Anemopsis californica **yerba mansa root**
Yerba mansa is a cooling, bitter herb and is a strong inflammation-mediating antimicrobial. It is used for upper respiratory infections, in particular for persistent sinus infections that are often resistant to any other treatment.

Yerba mansa is a berberine-containing herb, and is best taken as a tincture or powder. The tincture can be used, well diluted, for stubborn sinus infections.

Angelica archangelica **angelica root**
Angelica is a warming, bitter tonic herb, able to both stimulate and relax. So it is useful for weak digestion where there is bloating, heartburn, gastric fullness, pain and wind. It gently stimulates the liver and pancreas, helping digestion.

Angelica is seen as being both parasympatholytic and sympatholytic, calming an overactive sympathetic nervous system, which can shut down digestion and prevent relaxation; and also improving parasympathetic hyperactivity where there is poor digestion, sometimes with lots of mucus. It can also be used for respiratory mucus, promoting expectoration and clearing sinus congestion and for headaches caused by stress.

Materia Medica

Angelica is also used for vascular disease where there is poor circulation or intermittent claudication, maybe with headaches or migraines.[6]

A cold water infusion of the root can be used, using cold instead of boiling water, and infusing it overnight; or a decoction or any of the liquid extracts described below. Angelica is often mixed with cooling bitter herbs and aromatic herbs to make a digestive tonic formula.

The only time that bitters are contraindicated is when there are active gallstones that might be moved with them. Otherwise there are no contraindications.

Apium graveolens **celery**
Celery seed is an inflammation-mediating, diuretic and antispasmodic herb acting mostly on the digestive and urinary systems but also throughout the body as it is able to help inflammation and heat wherever it is found. So it might be helpful for gout, bladder inflammation or arthritic symptoms. It is seen as a regenerative herb for the kidneys and liver.[7]

It is also seen as a gentle sedative. Celery seed is specific for restlessness, sleeplessness, nervousness, anxiety and a brain 'debilitated from overwork or excitement', as well as a throbbing headache.[8]

It has been shown that *Apium graveolens* contains aglycones, which show potent inhibitory activity against LPS-induced inflammation.[9]

A review of studies found that celery, because of compounds such as caffeic acid, *p*-coumaric acid, ferulic acid, apigenin, luteolin, tannin, saponin and kaempferol, has powerful antioxidant characteristics to remove free radicals.[10]

Celery seed can be taken as tea or tincture, and it should be avoided in pregnancy. Celery as a vegetable is fine to be taken as food at any time.

Arctium lappa, **burdock root**
Burdock root is a cooling bitter, and bitters increase vagal tone as well as help digestion. Burdock root acts as an alterative, improving detoxification via the liver, skin, kidneys and lymph.

It is a herb useful to use in chronic ill health and especially where there are skin lesions or inflammation as well. It pairs well with dandelion root to improvs removal of toxins. It will be most helpful when body aches and

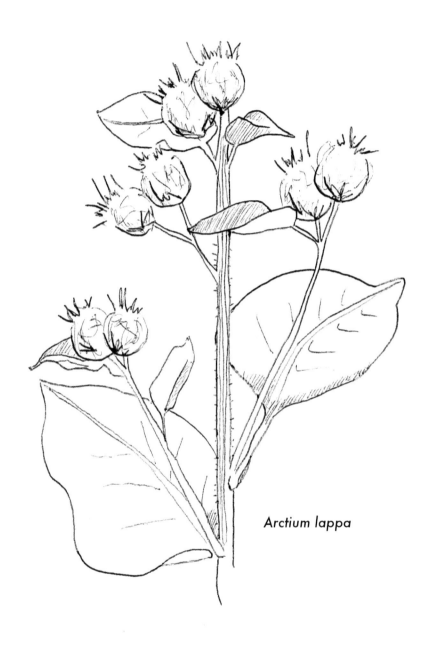

Arctium lappa

pains are worse for sitting still, and better for brisk movement. Burdock is a stimulating and restoring tonic for the liver, kidneys and pancreas, and is hypoglycaemic,[11] so is very useful in metabolic disease.

It is generally advisable to start with a low dose when taking burdock as it can provoke quite a strong detoxification reaction such as headaches, skin breakouts or nausea in those who have poor elimination systems. Traditionally it would be taken with dandelion in order to improve elimination and reduce these side effects.

Burdock root can be taken as tincture or decoction, and it makes a good coffee substitute when mixed with roasted dandelion root and a little cardamom or cinnamon and simmered as a decoction for ten to fifteen minutes. Suitable amounts would be one teaspoon each of burdock root and roasted dandelion root plus two cardamom pods and/or a pinch of cinnamon simmered in two cups of water. People who are often cold would do better not to use burdock root, it is very much a herb for those who run hot.

Armoracia rusticana **horseradish**
Horseradish is a heating, pungent root vegetable used medicinally as an inflammation mediator to clear mucous conditions of the respiratory tract such as bronchitis and sinusitis. It has been shown to inhibit the cyclooxygenase COX and lipoxygenase LOX pathways, and also to inhibit lipopolysaccharide (LPS) induced inflammation.[12]

Horseradish is most effective when taken fresh. It should be harvested in November and can be chopped and preserved for the year in cider vinegar if kept in the fridge.

Arnica montana **arnica flowers**
Arnica is a herb that is used either homeopathically or topically in nearly all cases as it has some toxicity. It is an inflammation mediating herb and is best known for tissue damage and bruising topically as an ointment or infused oil.

Arnica has a vascular effect and has been used, in very dilute quantities, in the same way as hawthorn, where it improves the blood supply through coronary vessels. It is said that the German writer and scientist Johann Wolfgang von Goethe (174–1832), to whom herbalists and plant lovers owe a debt for his research into botany, used arnica flower tea when he had angina pain owing to coronary arteriosclerosis.[13]
An alternative to arnica for bruising and tissue damage is daisy *Bellis perennis*, which has much less toxicity.

Inflammation

Artemisia vulgaris **mugwort**
Mugwort is a stimulating and decongesting bitter that acts as an inflammation mediator. It has an affinity for the uterus and liver, and is very effective when there is blood stagnation. It has a very long and extensive history of use as a menstrual and digestive herb and is recommended for polycystic ovarian syndrome (PCOS) and hyperandrogenism, which results in congestion, blood sugar imbalance and weight gain.[14]

Research has shown that mugwort has antioxidant, hypolipemic, hepatoprotective, antispasmodic, analgesic, antihypertensive, oestrogenic, cytotoxic, antibacteria, and antifungal effects [15]

Mugwort should not be taken in pregnancy or when breastfeeding, and is best not used long term as it has some toxicity.

Asclepias tuberosa **pleurisy root**
Pleurisy root is a stimulating and relaxing decongestant and cooling bitter and inflammation mediator that acts mainly on the lungs. It is helpful for hard, dry coughs, pleurisy and pneumonia. It also improves gastrointestinal, liver and kidney function.[16]

As a diaphoretic it relaxes peripheral capillaries and increases perspiration, cooling a hot and dry state. It is a very effective expectorant and is used in both acute and chronic respiratory conditions including asthma.

Pleurisy root is contraindicated in pregnancy.

Asparagus racemosus **wild asparagus or shatavari**
The Ayurvedic name shatavari means "she who has a hundred husbands". Shatavari is an adaptogen that is well respected as a herb for women of all ages, and is often used to aid fertility, lactation and menopause. It is inflammation mediating, immune modulating, moistening and cooling, and has an affinity for female reproductive organs as well as the bladder and digestive system.

It is known as a rejuvenative tonic particularly for women, but also useful for men. It is also hepatoprotective and cardioprotective and is used where there is neurodegeneration.[17]

Additionally It is also helpful for urinary system irritation and inflammation, and also for anxiety. It is very much a tonic herb.
It can be taken as a powder or a tincture and is safe for most situations, including pregnancy and breas feeding. the only time it is best not to take is if there is oestrogen induced fibrocystic breast disease.

Astragalus membranaceus **astragalus**
Astragalus is sweet, and somewhat warm and dry, and is an adaptogen, immunostimulant and tonic herb, which also acts on the cardiovascular system to reduce hypertension by vasodilation. As such it has multiple effects on inflammation throughout the body.

Astragalus is well respected as a liver and kidney protective and restorative herb.

In Chinese medicine astragalus is a spleen qi tonic, used for fatigue and weakness, and alongside chemotherapy to prevent immunosuppression and also to enhance the action of the chemotherapy. For this it is often used with milk thistle.

As an immunostimulant astragalus promotes the proliferation of immune cells, stimulates the release of cytokines, and affects the secretion of immunoglobulin and conduction of immune signals; it acts as an ant-tumour agent by enhancing immunity, inducing apoptosis of tumour cells and inhibiting the proliferation and transfer of tumour cells. It has been shown to be anti-aging; has antiviral effects; can regulate blood glucose in diabetics; and is lipid-lowering.[18]

The main contraindication for astragalus is that it should not be used when there is a lot of heat in the body, as in early stages of acute infection, for example. Astragalus should be used later, in the recovery stages when the strongest heat is past.

Azadirachta indica **neem**
Neem is a cooling bitter astringent herb mainly used for infections and inflammation. It is particularly useful as a liver protective and will also aid inflammatory arthritis and skin problems. It cools heat in its many forms, and reduces blood lipids and hypertension. Externally it is useful for skin and nail funga , parasitic and bacterial infections.
 Neem should be avoided internally in pregnancy or when breastfeeding; and is best taken short term.

Baptisia tinctoria **wild indigo**
Wild indigo is a strong alterative with affinity for the lymphatic system and lungs. It is very bitter and cooling, and is excellent as an antimicrobial and inflammation mediator, especially where there is infection with inflammation. It is indicated where there is liver and intestinal stagnation with damp heat. It was used extensively and successfully during typhoid epidemics in the nineteenth century.

Wild indigo is a strong herb and is best used short term or in small amounts in a formula with other herbs. Small doses (10 drops or so of 1:2 tincture) are stimulant and laxative, medium doses (2–30 drops –1.5ms) are anti-infective and cooling, and larger doses (more than 3ms) can be emetic and toxic.[19]

It can be used topically on skin infections or as a gargle for sore throats or infected tonsils.

Wild indigo is contraindicated in pregnancy.

Barosma betulina **buchu**
Buchu is a stimulating and diffusive ant-microbial herb that acts as an in-flammation mediator particularly for the kidneys and bladder, but also for any pelvic congestion. It is warming and astringent, and as such is useful where there is weakness and cold, damp conditions. This might include urinary frequency, chronic urinary infections and prostate congestion or chronic infection.

Buchu contains volatile essential oils, so if taking it as an infusion it is best to either make a cold infusion, or to use a lid so that condensed volatiles can re-enter the infusion.

It is not advised to use buchu for too long, on its own or when there is an acute infection. It makes a nice tea when mixed at a strength of about ten percent with other urinary system herbs such as *Althaea* or *Zea*.

Bellis perennis **daisy**
Daisy is a close relative of arnica *Arnica montana* and is as good as arnica for bruising and pain relief of injuries. It is better than arnica because it can also be used on open wounds, which is forbidden with arnica. Daisy has had a good reputation as a wound healing herb for a very long time – the Romans used daisy juice to treat sword and spear wounds[0]
Daisy has been used for inflammatory conditions as diverse as liver in-flammation, eye inflammation and painful joints and gout.[20]

Daisy can be used internally, except in pregnancy, as a tea or tincture, or externally as an ointment.

Berberis vulgaris **barberry root**
Barberry is a stimulant and alterative herb for the liver, gallbladder and digestion. It is bitter and cooling, and contains berberine, an alkaloid that

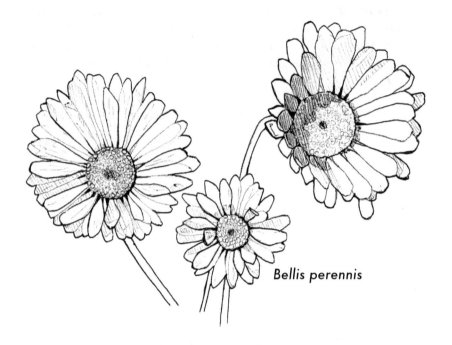

Bellis perennis

is also present in several other yellow roots (such as *Hydrastis canadensis*, *Anemopsis californica* and *Mahonia aquifolium)*, and which has been shown to normalise endothelial cell function and act as an anti-atherosclerotic that will protect the body from cardiovascular and metabolic disease. It has been shown to act as an inflammation mediator and as a hypotensive; and to reduce insulin resistance and hyperglycaemia [21]

Barberry is most useful where there is a great deal of heat and inflammation, with a red or coated tongue and a rapid pulse.[22]

It is an excellent mover for the digestive system, great for sluggish digestion and bowels, and for liver congestion. As an antimicrobial it is useful for any gut infections such as gastroenteritis, and liver infections such as hepatitis. It is contraindicated in pregnancy.

Boswellia serrata frankincense resin
Frankincense resin has been used for many generations in warmer climes to treat chronic inflammatory disease and pain. It is bitter and astringent and is a COX-2 inhibitor. Studies on boswellic acid, just one component of frankincense, have shown that it is able to modulate many different chronic inflammatory diseases – from cancer and diabetes, to asthma, in-

flammatory bowel disease and psoriasis. There are several boswellic acids, but all have shown the ability to inhibit the pro-inflammatory enzyme 5-lipoxygenase.[23]

It is recognised today as an antiarthritic, inflammation mediating, antihyperlipidaemic, antiatherosclerotic, analgesic and hepatoprotective herb.[24]

Boswellia was compared with valdecoxib, a non steroidal anti-inflammatory drug, in a randomised trial over six months of 66 patients with knee arthritis. Valdecoxib provided pain and stiffness relief within one month but its effects were lost as soon as treatment stopped. Boswellia took two months for most people to bring relief but its effects lasted one month after treatment stopped [25]

It enhances immunity and is also useful in autoimmune disease; it is also recommended for its meditative effect.[26]

The tincture tastes particularly vile, but frankincense can be taken as an aromatic water or as powder in capsules. Frankincense should be avoided in pregnancy.

Calendula officinalis **English or Pot marigold flowers**
Calendula is a wonderful healing herb that is inflammation-mediating, alterative, antiseptic, antispasmodic and vulnerary (healing to body tissue). It is useful to improve both lymphatic and liver function, especially where these are sluggish. It is warming and stimulating but also parasympathomimetic, able to help the body back into parasympathetic mode and relaxation.

Calendula petals can be taken as a tea, or tincture or as powder; or made into an infused oil to use topically. Calendula flowers make an excellent foot or hand bath for arthritic joints, and are even better with yarrow. They are very safe and have no contraindications.

Cannabis sativa, C. indica cannabis, CBD oil
Cannabidiol CBD oil is the legally available (in the UK) extract of cannabis that contains less than 0.2% tetrahydrocannabinol (THC), which is the psychoactive part of cannabis. CBD oil is not psychoactive.

Cannabis has been used for possibly thousands of years worldwide to treat pain, insomnia, anxiety, inflammation, epilepsy, nausea and vomiting. Cannabis as a whole plant is illegal in the UK, but CBD oil is legal and is a very popular and well-researched supplement.

Materia Medica   163

Generally CBD oil from *Cannabis sativa* is seen as the more stimulant of the two plants, but if taken during the day for pain or inflammation it also has a beneficial effect on sleep. CBD oil from *Cannabis indica* is mostly used for sleep issues, and so is generally taken in the evening, but is also fine during the day as its action is more relaxing than soporific.

CBD is a strong inflammation mediator and antioxidant, and it has been shown to have a beneficial effect on arthritic, cardiovascular, neurodegenerative, cancer and metabolic disease. In diabetes it has been shown to have a therapeutic effect on diabetic neuropathy, and has been shown to improve the overall health of diabetics.[27]

CBD has been shown to improve cognition in Alzheimer's disease by increasing two proteins, TREM2 and IL33, which are involved in clearing debris, including beta-amyloid plaque, in the brain. These proteins are decreased in Alzheimer's. CBD has also been shown to reduce IL6, which is pro-inflammatory.[28]

When taking CBD oil it is important to start with a low dose and build up slowly until the required effect is noticed. It is very safe with few side effects, but can affect liver clearance of medications so guidance must be sought before taking it alongside any medication.

Capsicum annuum cayenne fruit
Cayenne is a heating (very hot) stimulant and will clear sinuses or any mucous congestion of the upper respiratory tract. It is able to shock the vagus back into tone, which might be helpful after any trauma that might include blood loss or tachycardia. It is also indicated for any circulatory problem, including internal or external bleeding, which it is excellent at stopping. As it is so hot it is contraindicated for people who are already hot, however in an emergency as a single use it is fine.

It can be used as powder, fresh fruit or tincture. As an ointment it is excellent for skin pain where nerves are involved, for example when there is skin pain after shingles.

As with all strong herbs it is generally best to start with a very small amount and build up as needed.

Carbenia benedicta blessed thistle
Blessed thistle is a stimulating, bitter herb that acts as a decongestant particularly for a sluggish liver, but also for cerebrospinal circulation. It is said to be an autonomic nervous system balancer through hepatic regulation.[29]

Inflammation

Modern research has shown that blessed thistle has antidepressive, inflammation-mediating, antiseptic, cardiac and antimicrobial properties, and it contains many phenolic compounds, including ursolic acid, genistin, and isorhamnetin, which have been shown to be excellent inflammation mediators, antioxidants and antidiabetic agents.[30]

As a stimulating bitter it is also effective to improve digestion and it was a well-respected herb in the past when it was used as an emetic to expel poisons from the body.

Blessed thistle is also an impressive alterative, acting on all channels of elimination, from the skin, kidneys, liver, bowels and lungs. Matthew Wood considers it to be excellent at reducing high androgen levels, as seen in many common female hormonal imbalances, the hormone most difficult for the liver to detoxify. He specifies blessed thistle as being the herb to try for frontal headaches associated with the liver and digestion.[31]

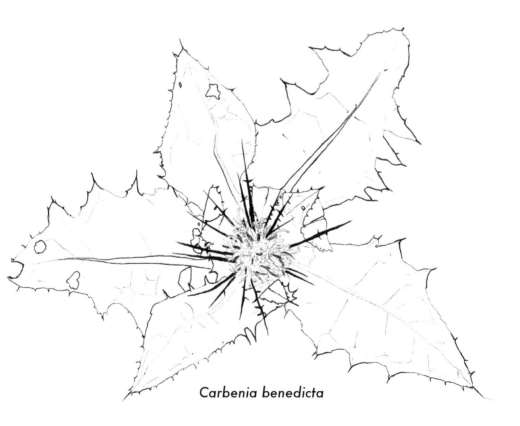

Carbenia benedicta

As a bitter it also helps to reset the vagus nerve, allowing better relaxation.

Blessed thistle is easiest to take as tincture, rather than a tea, as it is so bitter. The only time that bitters are contraindicated is when there are active gallstones that might be moved with them. Otherwise there are no contraindications.

Centaurium erythraea centaury
Centaury is a beautiful little pinky-red flowered herb that rivals gentian as one of the most bitter plants used medicinally. As a bitter it acts on the digestive system, including the gallbladder and liver, and is parasympathomimetic, aiding relaxation. It also stimulates pancreatic secretion, aiding blood sugar balance.

As it is so bitter it is best taken in drops as a tincture. The only time that bitters are contraindicated is when there are active gallstones that might be moved with them. Otherwise there are no contraindications.

Centella asiatica gotu cola
Gotu cola is a calming and cooling adaptogenic nervine tonic with a strong inflammation-mediating action on the whole system. It is able to balance the autonomic and central nervous systems,[32] and is used as a blood tonic and detoxifier for skin disorders, arthritis and autoimmune disease.

A review of clinical studies showed that gotu cola had extensive beneficial effects on neurological and skin diseases. The review found inflammation-mediating effects, antioxidative stress reduction, anti-apoptotic effects, and improvement in mitochondrial function. Looking at neurological disease, the pathogenesis of Alzheimer's disease and Parkinson's disease involve neuroinflammatory activities, oxidative stress, mitochondrial dysfunction, and dysfunction in brain-derived neurotrophic factor. The review found that all four aspects were improved by gotu cola.[33]

Gotu cola is useful for anxiety, insomnia, depression, brain fog and long-term illness or convalescence. It is also useful for wound healing topically.

It is best used as fresh leaf, but can be used as tincture or tea. As an adaptogen it is a very safe herb with no restrictions.

Chionanthus virginicus fringe tree
Fringe tree is a cooling, bitter and stimulating hepatic herb that promotes biliary and pancreatic secretions, improving tone and function of the liver,

Inflammation

gallbladder and pancreas. It is inflammation-mediating and antioxidant, and is a useful herb for blood sugar balance and pre-diabetic and diabetic states.

It has been used in the past as a specific for jaundice and for gallstones.[34] It is also specific for inflammatory digestive problems such as gastritis or irritable bowel, especially when poor digestion and liver function are involved.[35]

Fringe tree is best taken as powder or tincture.

The only time that bitters are contraindicated is when there are active gall-stones that might be moved with them. Otherwise there are no contraindications.

Cinnamomum spp. **cinnamon**
Cinnamon is warming and stimulating, and is commonly used to aid digestion. It also has a strong antimicrobial effect, and is an effective antibacterial and antifungal. Cinnamon has been recommended for diabetes and metabolic syndrome as a blood sugar- and lipid-reducing agent.

It is also useful as a circulatory stimulant so may be contraindicated where menstrual periods are heavy.

It is contraindicated in pregnancy, and is also very high in salicylates so caution is needed when there is any gut damage, and it is probably advisable not to take it long-term on its own.

Citrus aurantium fr. **bitter orange peel**
Bitter orange peel is bitter, sweet, antispasmodic and relaxing. It is a good digestive stimulant and is useful when there is any gas, bloating and pain. It relaxes smooth muscle and eases the pain of colic and dysmenorrhoea. It clears damp heat and reduces inflammation, particularly of the digestive tract.

It has been used as a stimulant for metabolism in diabetes and obesity, and is useful because it doesn't stimulate the cardiovascular system.[36] Bitter orange peel tastes good and can be used in decoction, tincture or aromatic water. As an essential oil (bergamot) it is helpful for massage of painful muscles. The aroma of the essential oil is very uplifting emotionally. Bergamot oil is a good inflammation-mediating oil as well as being antibacterial, so is useful for skin inflammation and infection.

Coriandrum sativum **coriander seed**
Coriander seed is a cooling aromatic herb that has been found to have many useful properties including antioxidant, digestive, antiseptic and inflammation-mediating. It has been shown to reduce LDL cholesterol and increase HDL cholesterol.[37]

Coriander seeds have been shown to have hypotensive effects by enhancing the interaction of calcium ions and acetylcholine, which relaxes blood vessel tension. Diuretic activity adds value to its use in hypertension.[38]

Coriander seed tastes good and can be used as much as desired in cooking. It is useful to stimulate digestion without being heating and can help with heartburn, indigestion, flatulence and diarrhoea. As a gargle it is helpful for throat infections, or as a wash for eye infections.

Corydalis spp. **corydalis root**
Corydalis is warming, bitter and stimulating. It is important in Chinese medicine for pain, and is a potent inflammation mediating herb as well as analgesic. Studies have been done on some of the alkaloids contained in corydalis, and they have been found to occupy opioid, cannabinoid and dopamine receptors.[39] It is a central nervous system depressant and useful for all kinds of pain; it can also be used to help sleep and anxiety.

Corydalis is best taken as powder or tincture. It is contraindicated in pregnancy.

Crataegus monogyna **hawthorn**
Hawthorn is the most well-known and well-used herb for the cardiovascular system. It is a cardiac and circulatory tonic, and is able to act as an antispasmodic and calming herb. It is the best herb for a nervous heart, where anxiety and palpitations are together and is recommended for degenerative and deficient conditions of cardiac function such as angina, weak or failing heart tissue, and any heart or circulatory disease including hypertension.

The berries are high in inflammation-mediating alkaloids and are also useful for inflammatory airways diseases.

The berries can be taken as a powder or in liquid form as a glycerate or tincture. The flowering tops are also good as a tea or tincture.

Curcuma longa **turmeric**
Turmeric has become very well known as an inflammation-mediating

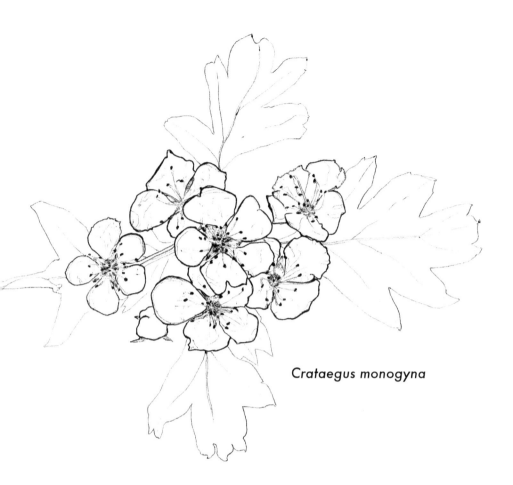

Crataegus monogyna

herb, but has had the unfortunate effect of creating an allergen when it is taken too much for too long. It is high in salicylates and, for some people, this has meant that it causes gut irritation and intolerance to other high-salicylate foods.

There is no doubt that it is a good inflammation-mediating herb (among many other attributes) but it should be taken with caution and not every day. Absorption is improved by taking it alongside black pepper *Piper nigrum*; this can be as powder in capsules, smoothie or in warm milk, or as a tincture.

Cynara scolymus **artichoke leaf**
Artichoke is a very bitter and cooling herb that is restorative and protective to liver and kidney function. It has been shown in clinical trials to reduce both total cholesterol and LDL cholesterol[40] and is a powerful antioxidant.

It is a useful addition to herbal formulae that aid digestive function. As it is a strong bitter it is best taken as a tincture.

The only time that bitters are contraindicated is when there are active gall-stones that might be moved with them. Otherwise there are no contraindications.

Dioscorea villosa **wild yam**
Wild yam is an excellent antispasmodic and relaxant herb, especially for the digestive system and liver. It acts on the autonomic nervous system to relax spasms and relieve irritation and pain, and is often used for colic-type pains as well as menstrual and birth pains.

It contains inflammation-mediating steroidal saponins and has been used traditionally in South America to treat arthritic conditions.

Wild yam is best taken as a powder or a tincture.

Echinacea purpurea, E. angustifolia **echinacea**
These are probably the best known of the immune-modulating herbs, and opinion is divided as to whether they should be used short- or long-term, and whether they cause flare-ups in those with autoimmune disease. Well-respected herbalists are on both sides of the argument.

As an immune-modulating herb, echinacea is able to increase immune status in resting immune cells so that a faster response occurs when needed; but when immune cells are overstimulated the immune response can be dampened to reduce symptoms.[41]

As well as being an excellent immunomodulant, echinacea is also inflammation-mediating and alterative, especially acting on the lymphatic system. It is therefore very useful in infections of all kinds to moderate symptoms and shorten infection duration. Numerous clinical studies testify to this, but it is important to take a high enough dose. The equivalent of about 1,000mg a day or 10ml of a 1:5 tincture is the minimum that should be used in acute infection.

Elettaria cardamomum **cardamom pods**
Cardamom pods are warming and aromatic, and often used to improve digestive function, particularly when digestion is weak or there are food allergies. Cardamom is also an excellent inflammation mediator acting on the digestive and respiratory systems.

Inflammation

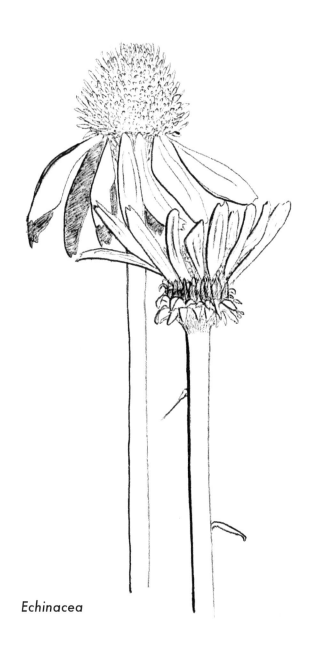

Echinacea

It has been shown to be very effective against *Porphyromonas gingivalis* and other bacteria involved in periodontitis and is able to inhibit biofilm formation.

Cardamom also significantly decreases secretion of inflammatory mediators secreted by lipopolysaccharide-stimulated macrophages, making it especially useful in chronic inflammation.[42]

Cardamom pods can be used in food, or made into a decoction or tincture.

Eleutherococcus senticosus **Siberian ginseng or eleuthero**
Eleuthero is an adaptogen and tonic herb. It is an immunostimulant, is able to regulate blood sugar and has a strong inflammation-mediating effect throughout the body. It has an affinity for the circulatory system and is useful for blood pressure regulation, atherosclerosis, and any circulatory insufficiency.[43]

It can be too stimulating for those who are very depleted, and may be better taken in the morning rather than later in the day. Eleuthero can be taken as tincture or powder.

Equisetum arvense **horsetail**
Horsetail is an inflammation-mediating herb and tonic, acting mostly on the kidneys and bladder, but also on connective tissue. It is helpful for cystitis, urethritis and prostate problems.

Horsetail contains a lot of silica, which is water soluble and is very useful to strengthen bones and other body tissues, so it is best made into a tea in a formula with other herbs.

Eucalyptus globulus, E. radiata **eucalyptus**
Eucalyptus is an excellent inflammation-mediating herb with a particular affinity for the respiratory system, where it is useful to clear phlegm, promote sweating and alleviate difficult respiration. It is also antiseptic.

Eucalyptus is used as a tea or as essential oil for colds, flu and all bronchial infections.

Eupatorium perfoliatum **boneset**
Boneset is an inflammation-mediating and diaphoretic herb that is cooling and bitter. It is very useful for upper respiratory tract infections, fevers and catarrh, and can relieve the aching muscles of viral infections. It is a herb that should be used short-term only as it contains some liver-toxic pyrrolizidine alkaloids.[44]

Boneset, made into an infusion, has a very long history of use for fevers, and was specific for malaria and dengue fever. It was introduced to Western herbalists via native Americans.

Given its potential toxicity it should be avoided by children, in pregnancy and where there is any liver disease.

Eupatorium purpureum gravel root

Gravel root is a tonic and inflammation-mediating herb for the kidneys and bladder, and is specifically used for conditions of congestion, infection, inflammation and gravel in that area.

Generally it is most useful where these conditions are chronic rather than acute. It is a very safe herb and can be taken as a decoction or tincture.

Euphrasia officinalis eyebright

Eyebright is an astringent and inflammation-mediating herb with an affinity for the eyes and upper respiratory tract. It is helpful to calm and cool irritated mucous membranes, especially when caused by seasonal allergies or infections.

A study has shown that eyebright can reduce UVB-induced photoaging in the eyes by alleviating oxidative stress, pro-inflammatory activity and cell apoptosis.[45]

Eyebright is mostly used as an infusion, especially when applied to eyes. There are no contraindications.

Foeniculum vulgare fennel seed

Fennel seed has an aniseed flavour and is sweet and warming to the digestive tract. It is an excellent digestive, relieving gas and digestive bloating, and the tea can be given to babies to alleviate colic. Fennel seed is also a useful inflammation mediator and expectorant, making it useful in respiratory infections and inflammation.

It appears that fennel seed can block the inflammatory processes induced by lipopolysaccharides, by regulating pro-inflammatory cytokine production, transcription factors and nitric oxide.[46]

As an infusion it can also be used as an eyewash to alleviate any inflammation of the eyes.

Fennel seed is contraindicated in pregnancy as it is a uterine stimulant.

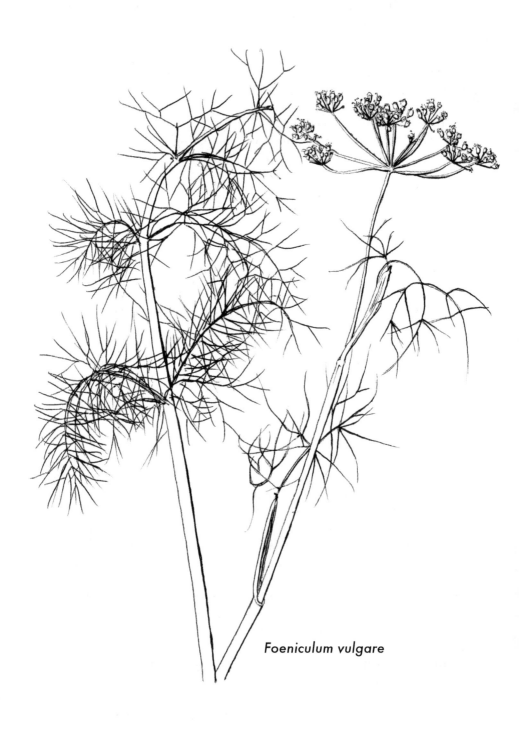

Foeniculum vulgare

Inflammation

Galium aparine **cleavers**

Cleavers acts on the lymphatic circulation and the kidneys to assist the removal of toxicity. It is cooling and will help irritation and inflammatory processes of the kidneys and bladder. Cleavers has been shown to stimulate immune cells as well as having antioxidant properties.[47]

Cleavers is a well-respected lymphatic alterative and is a very safe herb that can be taken long-term. It is best used fresh, and can be juiced or added to green smoothies. Otherwise it can be taken as tea or tincture. The tea can be made in the standard way or as a cold infusion by simply adding fresh herb to cold water and leaving it for several hours.

Ganoderma lucidum **Reishi mushroom, fruiting body, mycelium and spores**

Reishi mushroom is an adaptogen and is non-toxic and fairly gentle, helping the body to adapt to stress and changing conditions such as aging. It regulates as needed, so immunity, liver function, cardiovascular function, sleep or the need for alertness – all are upregulated or downregulated as needed by the body. A very clever fungus!

Many of the properties of reishi can be directly attributed to the lucideric and ganoderic acids, which are the main triterpenes present in ganoderma. These are inflammation-mediating, inhibit histamine release, are sedative, antihepatotoxic, antihypertensive, hypolipidaemic, antiviral and anticancer. They are present in the highest concentration in the spores rather than the fruiting body, although if this is all that is available then it will be fine. Triterpenes in general are soluble in oil or high alcohol content and not very soluble in water so are best taken as a powder or in special extracts.

Reishi has been reported to exhibit antioxidant, anti-inflammatory and analgesic effects with potential therapeutic benefits against a wide range of diseases, including hepatitis, hypertension, arthritis, bronchitis and malignancy.[48]

Reishi is calming, sedative and helps anxiety; it helps with insomnia and improves sleep quality. It has been used for withdrawal from addictive substances, and can reduce the effect of caffeine on the body.
It is a circulatory tonic, and can reduce high blood pressure (by inhibiting angiotensin converting enzyme (ACE), which allows blood vessels to dilate). It is also a heart tonic that helps vagal tone and improves the ability to relax.

It contains a five-alpha-reductase inhibiting agent that blocks testosterone conversion to dihydrotestosterone and reduces prostate enlargement. Its inflammation-mediating properties will help with arthritic pains; and its antihistamine properties will reduce allergic reactions.

Reishi is a very useful medicine for those with chronic fatigue. They need help with inflammation, immunity, fatigue, anxiety, insomnia despite fatigue, and brain function among other issues, but that help has to be gentle, not pushy.

Reishi spores and fruiting body are available as powder or in capsules, and the fruiting body is also available as a glycerate or tincture, both made by first decocting and then adding glycerine or alcohol respectively.

Gentiana lutea gentian
Gentian is intensely bitter, possibly one of the most bitter herbs available, and as such it is best taken in drop form as a tincture, or mixed into a formula where it forms just a small percentage.

Gentian is an excellent tonic for the digestive system, improving the digestive ability of the gut. As a flower essence it is helpful for those who doubt their own abilities, or doubt the path they are on, and it brings hope and optimism. This applies to the herb as well as the flower essence.

Gentian is very helpful for those whose digestion shuts down and appetite goes when emotions become labile. As a strong bitter it can really improve vagal tone, and often do it quickly, allowing relaxation when the body has become very tense. As such it is useful for panic attacks, hysteria, shock or intense anger.

Gentian is also inflammation-mediating – one study showed it could inhibit LPS-induced expression of TNF-alpha in macrophages.[49] It has also been shown to prevent endothelial inflammation, the root cause of cardiovascular disease.[50]

The only time that bitters are contraindicated is when there are active gallstones that might be moved with them. Otherwise there are no contraindications.

Ginkgo biloba ginkgo leaf
Ginkgo is a circulatory stimulant and inflammation-mediating herb that is able to target the nervous system, including the brain, lungs and cardiovascular system. It is useful for inflammatory conditions affecting the lungs such as asthma. Its effects on the brain arise from its antioxidant and inflammation-mediating actions.[51,52, 53] It is able to improve cerebral and

cardiovascular circulation, and it has a protective and strengthening effect on the vascular system.[54]

Many studies have looked to see if gingko is helpful in treating dementia and Alzheimer's disease, and the best conclusion that could be drawn is that gingko is more effective than placebo.[55] Alzheimer's disease and dementia are both diseases of neuroinflammation, and while gingko is always going to help with this, if factors causing inflammation are not ad-

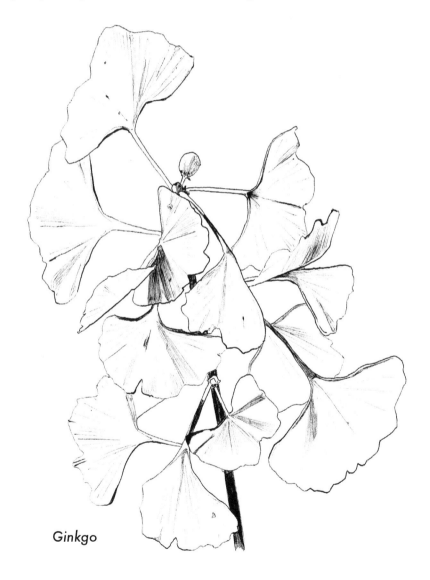

Ginkgo

dressed – with diet, supplements, meditation and so on – then no single herb is going to make any headway.

However, if ginkgo was put alongside measures to reduce neuroinflammation, it should have a good chance to improve the disease.

Gingko can be taken as a tea or a tincture. The only contraindication for gingko is alongside anticoagulant medication, when care should be taken.

Glechoma hederacea ground ivy aerial parts
Ground ivy is a common wild flower, easily identified and harvested. It is most commonly used to clear catarrhal conditions of the head, especially when the ears and nose are involved, but also for any lung congestion. Modern research has confirmed that it is a strong antioxidant and inflammation mediator.[56]

Ground ivy is generally seen as a very safe herb without contraindications, and can be taken as an infusion, tincture or glycerate.

Glycyrrhiza glabra liquorice
Liquorice is a very widely used herb, partly because its sweet taste is useful to improve the palatability of other herbs. It has been used as a medicinal herb for thousands of years and has been well researched. It is an adaptogen and is able to restore and regulate the hypothalamic–pituitary–adrenal axis.

Liquorice is useful for all conditions of inflammation and irritability of most mucous membranes of the body, including the digestive and respiratory tracts. It has been recognised that liquorice is able to act in a steroid-like manner, and it seems that this is because it inhibits the breakdown of corticosteroids in the body, thereby potentiating the anti-inflammatory effects of cortisol and ACTH.

This means that liquorice is useful in helping withdrawal from steroid medication. Unlike steroid medication, which will suppress adrenal function, liquorice will restore it. As an adaptogen, liquorice is able to increase cortisol when needed, and also decrease it if that needs to happen. Liquorice will balance adrenal hormones.

Liquorice is also excellent for all kinds of allergic reactions, and is also a good antiviral herb.

Unfortunately, it can also enhance aldosterone, which can create high blood pressure, so liquorice is contraindicated where there is already hypertension, and it should not be taken in large amounts long-term by anyone.

Grifola frondosa **maitake**
Maitake is a medicinal fungus, and is rich in beta-glucans, which are excellent immune modulators. It has been shown to have good inflammation-mediating, anticancer and anti-allergic properties.[57]

Maitake can improve insulin resistance and overall blood sugar control.[58] Maitake can be eaten, or it can be processed into powders and taken as a supplement. It appears to have no contraindications.

Gymnema sylvestre **gurmar**
Gurmar translates to 'sugar destroyer' in Hindi, which refers to the fact that it helps to reduce sugar cravings, and balance blood sugar levels. It is said to be one of the best remedies for diabetes.[59]

Gurmar has been shown to be effective in metabolic syndrome, reducing body weight, body mass index and LDL cholesterol levels.[60]

It also has inflammation-mediating properties especially when inflammation affects the liver or pancreas.

The main caution for gurmar is alongside blood sugar-reducing medication such as insulin – it is important to carefully monitor blood sugar.

Hemidesmus indicus **sariva**
Sariva, also known as Indian sarsaparilla, is an excellent antioxidant and inflammation mediator that also protects the liver, kidneys, heart and nervous system. It also acts as a hormone balancer and antidepressant.

It is particularly useful for inflammatory skin diseases and autoimmune disease, acting to calm and cool an overactive immune system.[61,62]

Sariva can be taken as powder or tincture.

Humulus lupulus **hops**
Hops are cooling, bitter and calming. They can help with anxiety, irritability and insomnia; they are also good where there is sluggish digestion or liver function alongside inflammation and heat.

Traditionally a hops pillow has been used to help insomnia – with appar-

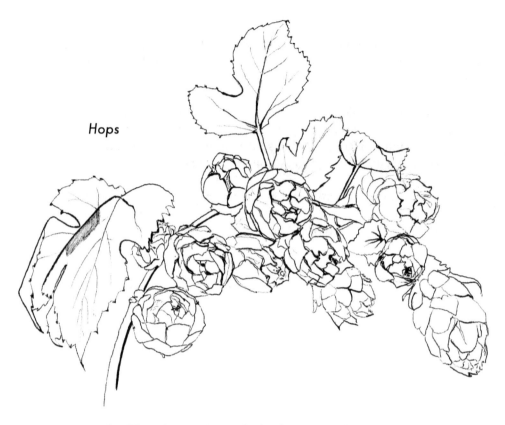

Hops

ent success for King George III and Abraham Lincoln. Hops are most successfully used for individuals who have intense personalities and strong emotions, and who are hot and easily angered. Hops can also be helpful in the relief of pain, especially when pain is in the head such as headache or toothache.[63]

Hops act as inflammation mediators particularly where that is needed for skin or digestion.[64]

Hops are contraindicated where there is depression, and, because they are phyto-oestrogenic, they are also contraindicated with oestrogen-sensitive cancers.

Hops can be taken brewed into beer, made into an infusion or as a tincture.

Hydrastis canadensis **goldenseal root**
Goldenseal is a cold, strong bitter with a tonic and inflammation-mediating effect on mucous membranes. It is restorative for all membranes and digestive organs, and may be used where there is inflammation, infection or stagnation in the liver, intestines and pancreas. It is also excellent

for infection or inflammation in the eyes or mouth. Berberine is one the most bioactive alkaloid constituents in goldenseal, and a review of studies showed numerous therapeutic effects for goldenseal including as an antimicrobial, anti-inflammatory, hypolipidemic, hypoglycemic, antioxidant, neuroprotective (anti-Alzheimer's disease), cardioprotective and gastrointestinal protective.[65]

Goldenseal should be taken short-term only, up to about 4 weeks, and should be avoided in pregnancy or when breastfeeding. It is generally taken as a tincture or powder, in small doses as part of a formula.

Hypericum perforatum St John's wort, aerial parts in flower
St John's wort is a cooling, astringent, inflammation-mediating and restorative herb. Its main action is on the nervous system, but it also acts on the liver and topically on the skin. St John's wort is above all a relaxing tonic herb for anxiety, restlessness and depression. It is also antiviral and as such, helpful for herpes both topically and internally.

It can also be used as a flower essence for depression, especially when linked with sunlight deprivation. As a flower essence it is perfect for hypersensitive people who are often overly affected by environmental stress or immune-related illness.

St John's wort has an ability to interact with the cytochrome P450 enzymes in the liver and intestinal lining that are used to metabolise many substances in the body. In particular, drug medications are very commonly metabolised by this system, and St John's wort will affect the absorption, metabolism and excretion of many drugs. Hence it is important not to take St John's wort at the same time as most prescribed medications, especially those that are very dose dependent. This is really a herb whose internal use is best prescribed by a herbalist, unless no medications are being taken.

However, it is fine to use topically for skin and nerve treatment. If no medications are being taken it is generally used as tincture or powder.

(See illustration on following page)

Inula helenium elecampane root
Elecampane is a warming, bitter and stimulating alterative, and potentially an adaptogen. It is most often used for inflammatory problems of the lungs where it has excellent tonic and inflammation-mediating actions. Elecampane is also an excellent antimicrobial and antiparasitic herb. It is

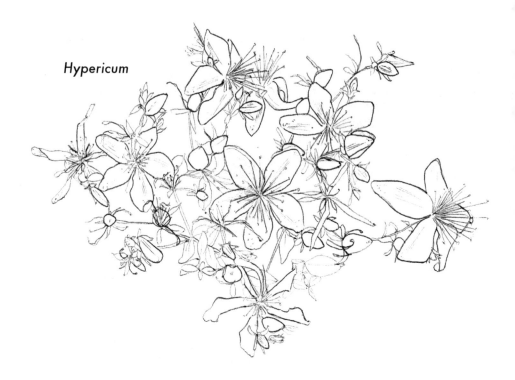

Hypericum

specific where there is yellow or green mucus, indicating bacterial infection.[66]

Elecampane was used in the past for conditions known as 'elfshot', where someone was so completely depleted that it was felt that they must have been shot by elves as there was no other explanation. This we would know today as chronic fatigue. Elfshot was also linked with sharp muscle pains from elf arrows, which we might today see as fibromyalgia.

Elecampane has a positive effect on the immune system, but is not over-stimulating, and is also good as an alterative, moving stagnation, particularly in the lungs, but also in the digestive tract.

Elecampane should be avoided in pregnancy as it also has an action on the uterus.

Elecampane can be taken as tincture or powder, or the fresh root can be cut into thin slices and candied in sugar.

Iris versicolor **iris or blue flag root**
Iris root is a cooling, bitter alterative that acts on the lymphatic and diges-

Inflammation

tive system. It is often used to improve elimination, especially when the skin, lymph and liver need improved function. So inflammatory skin conditions, and inflammatory liver and pancreas conditions as well as biliary and pancreatic insufficiency all benefit from the use of blue flag.

Blue flag should be taken in small doses, short-term, if taken on its own. However, as a small part of a formula it is much safer.

Juglans nigra walnut

The leaves, green hulls and black hulls of walnut are the parts used medicinally, and when the green hulls in particular are handled the hands will turn black as the iodine content is quite high. This has meant that black walnut is a very useful herb when the thyroid gland is underactive, and it has also been used for goitre.

Walnut is astringent, bitter and cooling, and acts as an alterative, especially on the lymphatic and digestive systems. Walnut is most useful to treat digestive problems when there is damp and stagnation. It is an excellent antibacterial and antifungal agent, especially for the skin or digestive system.

Walnut kernels also have significant inflammation-mediating properties,[67] and are especially good from a nutritional point of view.

Green walnuts can be used to make a delicious traditional liqueur called nocino, a slightly bitter drink that is a good digestive tonic. This is usually made in May or June, with whole unripe walnuts before they form a hard shell inside the green hull.

Leonurus cardiaca motherwort, aerial parts in flower

Motherwort is a cooling, astringent, bitter and antispasmodic nervine most often used for its action on the heart and the liver. It is very commonly used for menopausal hot flushes, especially when they are accompanied by palpitations, anxiety and insomnia, although in some women it can cause menstrual flooding.

It is equally useful for any situation where there is tachycardia or palpitations, including hyperthyroidism. It is useful premenstrually for any nervous or muscle tension causing dysmenorrhea.

Motherwort is useful for insomnia of menopause, especially when this occurs with palpitations and anxiety. A study of the effects of motherwort on endothelial tissue showed antioxidant action, increased production of

Materia Medica

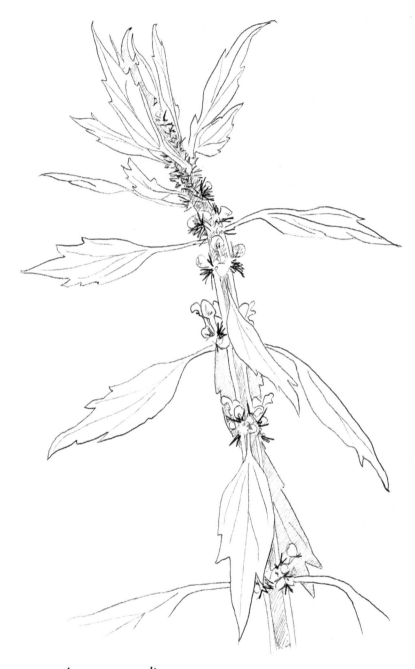

Leonurus cardiaca

Inflammation

nitric oxide (which improves endothelial function, and inhibits platelet aggregation), and an overall inflammation-mediating effect.[68]

As it is very bitter it is best taken as a tincture. It is not advised to use it during pregnancy.

Linum usitatissimum **linseed or flaxseed**
Linseed has been used for thousands of years as a cooling, inflammation-mediating and demulcent mucilagenous herb. It was used by Hippocrates, Dioscorides, Ibn Sina and Galen, and is a very safe herb.

It is useful for any inflammatory problems of the respiratory or digestive tract and can be helpful for both constipation and diarrhoea. Externally it makes a good poultice for any skin pain or inflammation.

When ground and mixed with water, linseed is able to absorb a lot of water and become very gloopy, so if it is to be taken internally it's best to mix it with water and drink it quickly. A good amount of linseed for internal use would be 1–2 tablespoons.

Lobelia inflata **lobelia, aerial parts in and after flowering**
Lobelia is a restricted herb (i.e. restricted to herbalists) but is one of the best warming antispasmodic and pain-relieving herbs in the Western materia medica.[69] It is very useful as an antispasmodic herb for coughing, especially dry and tickly spasmodic coughs. It is also an expectorant, which may be helpful for thick catarrhal lung conditions.

Lobelia also eases any breathing difficulties by relaxing lung, throat and chest muscles as well as the nervous system. Lobelia has an affinity to the vagus nerve,[70] and is able to relax the sympathetic nervous system and return the body to parasympathetic dominance.

As lobelia is a strong herb, and everyone's tolerance of it is different, it should only be taken in drop doses, and is best taken as a single herb so that the dose can be tailored exactly to the individual. The drops can be taken as needed, though. If too much is taken the likely outcome is first nausea, and then vomiting, so it is good to stop taking it for a while at the first sign of nausea.

There are contraindications for lobelia, so it should only be prescribed by a herbalist. It is also contraindicated in pregnancy, although it has been used historically to prevent miscarriage.

Lycopus europaeus **gypsywort**
Gypsywort is a cooling, bitter and relaxing herb used mostly for any condition where the pulse is rapid and the cardiovascular system is working overtime. This might be in hyperthyroidism, tachycardia or menopausal palpitations. It will relieve the tension and anxiety created by the cardiovascular system.

It has been shown to be inflammation-mediating,[71] and also has an impact on the thyroid gland. It appears to increase T4 excretion, thus improving symptoms of hyperthyroidism.[72]

It may not be useful in hypothyroidism as it may be able to suppress the thyroid further, and should also be avoided in pregnancy and breastfeeding.

Mahonia aquifolium **Oregon grape root**
Oregon grape is a berberine-containing alterative herb that is bitter, cold and liver-stimulating. It increases secretion from the digestive tract, thus improving digestion and assimilation. It is also a powerful antimicrobial.

Overall it improves metabolism and elimination, and is very useful for inflammatory skin diseases that benefit from improved body function. It is very similar to *Berberis vulgaris* (see above) but is more useful when the body is dry, secretions are low, and mucus is thick and unable to move.[73]

It has inflammation-mediating and antioxidant properties.[74]

As a bitter Oregon grape root is contraindicated when there are active gallstones that might be moved. It is also contraindicated in pregnancy, and should be taken with caution in hyperthyroid conditions.

Marrubium vulgare **white horehound**
White horehound is a stimulating bitter herb that has been used for many generations as a cough and lung remedy. It is a good expectorant and tonic for mucous membranes and has been shown to have antioxidant and inflammation-mediating properties.[75] It is effective against all kinds of coughs, sore throats and catarrh. As a stimulating bitter it will also have a beneficial effect on sluggish or weak digestion. White horehound is best avoided in pregnancy.

Matricaria chamomilla **German chamomile**
While it is a different plant, the medicinal actions of this chamomile and Roman chamomile *Anthemis nobilis*, are pretty much the same.

Chamomile has been used for generations as an infusion taken for tension, digestive pain and insomnia. It is antispasmodic, bitter, inflammation-mediating and cooling, acting on the digestive and nervous systems to relax and calm the whole body.

One study found that chamomile acts on the COX-2 pathway to mediate inflammation in a similar way to non steroidal anti-inflammatory drugs.[76]

It has been used for babies (of all ages) who are cross, whining and peevish, demanding attention and maybe irritated by teething or just simply irritated or out of sorts.[77] People who do well with chamomile tend to be those who tell all about their troubles, and probably overdramatise them – and if they try and eat while agitated they will end up bloated and in pain.

This is the herb to try first as a tea (maybe with ginger) for most cramping digestive pains as well as earache, toothache, headache, menstrual pain and nightmares. Chamomile has an affinity for the vagus nerve and will help to improve its tone.

When chamomile is the right herb it will create a feeling of calm and relaxation, and easy and prolonged sleep.

Both chamomiles can also be used as tea, tincture or essential oils.

Melissa officinalis **lemon balm leaf**
Lemon balm is a cooling, and sedative nervine, antispasmodic herb acting on the whole body. It is useful where there is anxiety, palpitations, rapid pulse, high blood pressure and digestive problems.

Lemon balm is also a good antioxidant and inflammation-mediating herb.

It has been shown to have a similar effect as atorvastatin on high LDL cholesterol levels, and has been recommended as a prevention of cardiovascular disease in diabetics, who also benefit from positive changes in blood sugar control, lipid profile, inflammation and hypertension when given lemon balm for 12 weeks.[78]

Lemon balm is a very safe herb, often used as a tea made from the leaves, which are especially good when made with fresh lemon balm.
Lemon balm should be used with caution in pregnancy as it is a mild uterine stimulant, and in untreated hypothyroidism as it may be able to block the conversion of thyroid hormone thyroxine to T3. This latter action is useful in treating hyperthyroidism, however.

Mentha piperita **peppermint leaf**

Peppermint is unusual because it is a stimulating and warming herb that tastes and acts in a cooling manner. This apparent paradox can be explained by its menthol content – menthol cools by opening skin pores and relaxing peripheral circulation, which warms by improving circulation. This makes peppermint a useful diaphoretic herb for use in a fever as it promotes sweating. It also helps to open blocked sinuses, and treat sinus headaches.

Peppermint is also antispasmodic and is very helpful for digestive colic and intestinal spasms – for some people. Others it doesn't help because peppermint is high in salicylates, hence anyone sensitive to salicylates might well find it causes heartburn. However, for those who can tolerate peppermint, it is also a useful antioxidant, inflammation-mediating and also antiviral herb.[79]

Peppermint is best taken as fresh leaf made into an infusion, but it can also be made from dried leaf, or can be used as essential oil.

Ocimum sanctum **holy basil, tulsi**

Holy basil is an adaptogen and tonic herb that has been used in India for many generations. It is greatly revered in Ayurveda as an elixir of life, being known as 'the incomparable one' and 'the Queen of herbs'. Daily consumption of holy basil is said to prevent disease, and promote general health, wellbeing and longevity.

Many studies have been done on holy basil, and it has been found to be antioxidant, inflammation-mediating, immunomodulating and antimicrobial; to protect against metabolic syndrome by normalising blood sugar and blood pressure; to protect against pollution and heavy metals; to protect against physiological stress through positive effects on memory and cognitive function, anxiety and depression. In short, there isn't much it can't do.[80]

It is best avoided during pregnancy, breastfeeding and in thyroid disease. Holy basil makes a very palatable infusion, and is excellent as a fresh herb. It can be grown very easily as an annual in the UK with a little protection.

Panax ginseng **Asian ginseng**

Asian ginseng is a highly prized herb, and is an adaptogen and tonic herb with a strong reputation for conferring energy, stamina and longevity. The many studies that have been done on it have shown that Asian ginseng

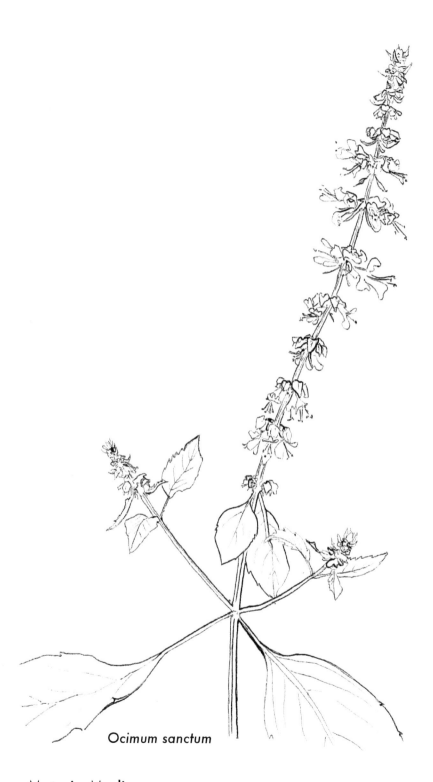

Ocimum sanctum

is excellent at maintaining homeostasis of the immune system, and is an excellent herb for conditions of chronic inflammation.[81]

It should not be used for acute inflammation or where there is excess heat or hypertension. It is also sometimes too strong for women, and is often better suited to the male constitution. If headaches result then it is the wrong herb for that person.

Phytolacca decandra poke root

Poke root is a powerful alterative with particular affinity for the lymphatic system, and is also an immune stimulant and inflammation mediator. It is especially indicated where there are hard or swollen lymph nodes or fibrocystic breast disease.

As it is so strong it is important to take only a low dose, and to stop or reduce the herb if any side effects such as digestive irritation or headaches are experienced. It should be avoided in pregnancy or breastfeeding, and avoided in kidney disease. It is best taken as a tincture.

Pimpinella anisum aniseed

Aniseeds are sweet, warming, relaxing and stimulating to the lungs, heart and digestive system. Aniseed has been found to relieve pain in dysmenorrhea, and in diabetic patients it showed hypoglycaemic and hypolipidaemic effects.[82]

Aniseed can be used as a culinary herb, as a long infusion or as tincture.

Piper nigrum black pepper

Black pepper is a pungent, heating aromatic spice that improves absorption and bioavailability of foods and medications, in particular curcumin from turmeric. It warms and stimulates the digestive system and has been shown to be antioxidant, inflammation-mediating, antitumour, antimutagenic and antimicrobial.[83]

Black pepper is useful in chronic inflammatory states, but less so where inflammation is acute and the body is hot.

Plantago lanceolate, P. major plantain

Plantain is one of the most useful first aid plants and can be found growing in most parts of the world at most times of the year. It is cooling, moistening, antiseptic (when fresh), antihistamine, and inflammation-mediating.[84]

It is also an excellent drawing agent and can be used on dirty wounds and abscesses to draw out infection and dirt; it has been used similarly for poisonous spider and snake bites, for tooth abscesses, and all types of bites and stings. It is also useful for relieving inflammation and irritation of the upper respiratory tract and lungs.

Plantain is best used as a fresh poultice for topical use, with well-chopped or chewed leaves applied to the skin. Or it can be added to a green smoothie, made into an infusion or tincture. All these preparations are most effective with fresh leaf if available.

Polygonum cuspidatum **Japanese knotweed**
Japanese knotweed is a herb that has been used for generations by traditional Chinese medicine as a treatment for many inflammatory diseases, but it has become notorious in Europe and North America for its invasive growth.

It is an important source for resveratrol, a supplement used as an inflammation mediator and hepatoprotective. It appears that the European Japanese knotweed contains lower concentrations of resveratrol than the Chinese plant.[85]

Japanese knotweed is cold and bitter, and has been shown to reduce blood sugar levels and inhibit COX-2. It is recognised as a useful antimicrobial in the treatment of Lyme disease and its co-infections, where its ability to protect the endothelium is important, as is its ability to reduce inflammation and cross the blood–brain barrier to reduce neuroinflammation.

It is also a strong inhibitor of cytokine storms in infection and is specific for bartonella as well as Lyme infection.[86]

Japanese knotweed is contraindicated in pregnancy, and should not be used with blood-thinning medication.

Prunella vulgaris **selfheal**
Selfheal was once seen as one of the best wound-healing herbs but is now more generally used to clear heat and mediate inflammation, especially circulatory. It is particularly useful for hypertension associated with heat, or fevers associated with infection. It acts as a lymphatic alterative and in China it is used for its antitumour properties.[87]

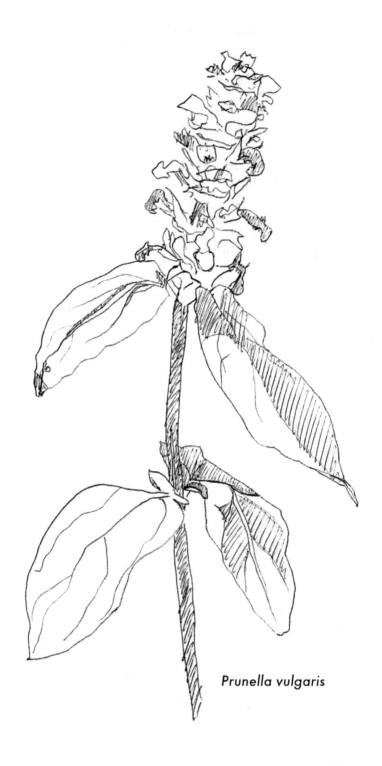

Prunella vulgaris

Inflammation

Selfheal is a very common plant that can be easily identified and harvested, and can be taken as infusion or tincture. There are no contraindications.

Rhodiola rosea **roseroot**
Rhodiola is astringent and sedative, but also increases physical and mental stamina and is adaptogenic and inflammation-mediating. It is used for depression and acute anxiety states.

Several studies have shown a protective effect on the heart as well as benefits for arrhythmia, hypertension and atherosclerosis.[88] It is able to cross the blood–brain barrier, reduce neuroinflammation, and act as a neuro-protective agent.[89] Clinical research has also shown benefits with fatigue, exhaustion and lack of concentration.[90]

It is easiest to take as powder or tincture, and its astringency is the only consideration for caution; if someone is already very dry, maybe with constipation, it isn't the best herb to take.

Rosa canina **dog rose**
Traditionally all parts of the rose have been used medicinally, but the hips and petals are the most commonly used. Rosehips are high in vitamin C as well as antioxidants, both of which make it useful as an inflammation mediator, particularly useful for arthritis.[91]

The petals are also effective for inflammation – both acute and chronic – of skin, respiratory tract, digestion and joints. Rose is an excellent women's tonic and hormone regulator, owing to its ability to lift the spirits and act on the liver.

Rose has no contraindications, and can be taken as infusion, powder, aromatic water or tincture.

Rumex crispus **yellow dock root**
Yellow dock root is a cooling, stimulating bitter that works as an alterative on the lymphatic, liver and digestive systems. It is useful for inflammation and overactivity in the digestive system indicated by acid reflux, heartburn, excess saliva and strong appetite. The bowels may be loose or constipated.

Redness of facial skin and a long, pointed red tongue are both indicators for yellow dock root.[92] Yellow dock root is useful in all conditions of chronic inflammation where the liver, bowels and lymph need their function enhanced to clear stagnation and remove toxins.[93]

Yellow dock root can be taken as a powder or as tincture, and is safe when used in moderation.

Salvia miltiorrhiza **red sage or danshen**
Red sage is a cooling bitter herb with an affinity for the heart and liver. It is seen as a blood-moving herb so is useful where there is stagnation.

Red sage is an important herb in the traditional Chinese materia medica where it is used in particular for cancer and cardiovascular disease. It is inflammation-mediating, antioxidant and antimicrobial,[94] and has been shown to be particularly effective at improving endothelial function, reducing antioxidative stress, reducing the risk of vascular blockage, inhibiting inflammation as well as regulating lipid metabolism, a combination often seen in metabolic syndrome and diabetes.[95]

Red sage is contraindicated alongside anticoagulant medication and in pregnancy.

Salvia officinalis **sage leaf**
Sage is an interesting herb, and its properties depend largely on its method of preparation. So a hot tea is used as a stimulant to sweating, salivation and internal secretions, while a cold tea will decrease secretions, including sweating, salivation, mucus formation and lactation.[96]

Sage is an excellent antimicrobial and is useful as a gargle for throat and mouth infections. It has been shown to be a strong antioxidant and inflammation mediator, and to act as an antidepressant and improve cognitive function in those with Alzheimer's disease.[97]

Sage is seen as rejuvenative and as a tonic herb in traditional Western and Ayurvedic herbal medicine, and is useful for fatigue, lowered immunity and nervous depletion.[98] It is also a useful digestive herb, used for indigestion, nausea, flatulence and any inflammation of the digestive tract.

There are some cautions with sage as it contains thujones, which can be toxic to some people. Indications of toxicity will often appear first as a headache, so this is a sign to discontinue sage. Generally sage is best taken short-term. It should also be avoided in pregnancy or breastfeeding.

Salvia rosmarinus (formerly *Rosmarinus officinalis*) **rosemary herb**
Rosemary is a warming, astringent, stimulating herb acting on most areas of the body. It stimulates the metabolism, improves circulation, digestion and liver function. It acts as an antispasmodic and can be very helpful for headaches and muscle tension.

Rosemary has inflammation-mediating, antioxidant, antimicrobial, anti-proliferative and protective functions,[99] and has been shown to be an effective antiviral against the COVID-19 virus.[100]

Rosemary warms the heart and mind, and lifts the spirits. It is useful for premenstrual syndrome with depression and painful periods, and for depression with cold, mental stupor, shyness and complacency, low self-esteem and fearfulness.

Rosemary can be taken as tea or tincture, or used topically as an essential oil for painful joints and muscles.

Sambucus nigra **elderflower and berry**
The elder tree is traditionally a source of many medicines – so much so that Charlemagne, an emperor in Europe around the year 800 CE, decreed that an elder should be planted by every household to provide medicine – from its leaves, flowers, berries and bark.[101]

These days we mostly use the flowers and berries as a very effective flu and cold remedy, as well as for seasonal allergies. The flowers have diaphoretic, decongestant and expectorant properties, and the berries are antiviral, antioxidant and inflammation-mediating.

The berries may also be an effective remedy for diabetes, obesity and metabolic syndrome as they have been shown to improve glucose and lipid metabolism.[102]

Elder berries and flowers make a very palatable syrup or glycerate, as well as an infusion or tincture. Anyone sensitive to salicylates should avoid elder.

Schisandra chinensis **schisandra**
Schisandra is an adaptogenic, inflammation-mediating, antioxidant herb with anticancer and antidiabetic effects. It has been shown to improve insulin resistance by inhibiting inflammation. It is able to improve cognitive behavioural function,[103,104] and has shown a protective role in neurodegenerative disease including stroke, dementia and depression.[105]

Schisandra 'calms the mind, lifts the spirits and aids memory, concentration and learning ability'.[106] It can also inhibit inflammatory bowel disease by regulating the composition and metabolism of gut microbiota[107] and is well recognised as a herb that both protects the liver and improves its function.

Schisandra is best taken as a decoction or tincture, and is contraindicated in pregnancy and where there is acute infection.

Scrophularia nodosa figwort

Figwort gets its Latin name from scrofula, which was the name given to swollen, hard and painful lymph nodes arising from infection, sometimes tubercular, and a stagnant lymphatic system. This is sometimes associated with acne too.

Figwort is bitter and cooling and clears heat and damp; it is an excellent lymphatic alterative, which also acts as an antifungal and antibacterial agent, and is inflammation-mediating. It will also help with other elimination systems in the body, improving bowel, liver and bladder function.

Figwort is often used for inflammatory skin disease as well as lymphatic congestion. It is best taken as a tincture or powder.

Scutellaria baicalensis Baikal skullcap

Baical skullcap root is cooling and bitter and possesses anticancer, antiviral and inflammation-mediating properties. It is able to inhibit cytokine production, reducing inflammation.[108]

It also has antiviral, antitumour, antioxidant and antibacterial effects, and can be used to treat respiratory tract infections, pneumonia, colitis, hepatitis and allergic diseases. It is very useful in reducing histaminic allergic reactions.[109]

Baical skullcap has been found to improve insulin resistance and improve a fatty liver through inhibition of inflammation.[110] It is useful for stress-related circulatory problems, including hypertension.

Baical skullcap should be avoided in the first three months of pregnancy and taken with caution alongside anticoagulant and hypoglycaemic medication.

Scutellaria lateriflora skullcap

Skullcap is a bitter, antispasmodic and cooling herb with a great affinity for the nervous system. It is used as a sedative and calming nervine and tonic herb for the brain and nervous system, and is particularly used for restlessness, irritability and agitation from any cause.

It is also inflammation-mediating and can be helpful as a pain reliever and hypotensive, especially if these conditions are associated with tension.

Skullcap can be taken as a tea or tincture and has no contraindications.

Serenoa repens **saw palmetto berry**
Saw palmetto is a sweet, warm and stimulating herb that is most commonly used for prostate enlargement, benign and malignant, and male infertility and impotence. It is also used for female infertility and amenorrhoea.

Saw palmetto is a plant native to the Southern USA, and in the eighteenth century it was noticed that livestock feeding on the berries grew heavier and stronger, so people decided to try it out. It is an excellent herb to strengthen and improve muscle density, especially in the elderly male.[111]

Saw palmetto should be avoided in pregnancy, and used with caution alongside anticoagulant medication. It is generally taken as a powder or tincture.

Silybum marianum **milk thistle seed**
Milk thistle is an excellent liver herb, sweet and bitter, warming and stimulating, and has been shown to protect the liver from damage by drugs, alcohol, pollution and chemicals. It protects the liver and also enhances its function.

Its hepatoprotective activity is unique and acts in different ways, including antioxidant and inflammation-mediating activities and stimulation of liver regeneration. This makes it an excellent herb for hepatitis. However, it also does more – milk thistle has also been found to have renal protective, hypolipidemic and anti-atherosclerosis qualities, and to stimulate cardiovascular protection and prevention of insulin resistance, especially in cirrhotic patients, cancer and Alzheimer's prevention.[112]

Milk thistle seed can be used in a pepper grinder to sprinkle on food, or it can be taken as a powder or tincture.

Solidago virgaurea **goldenrod**
Goldenrod is a cooling, astringent herb with an affinity for the upper respiratory tract and urinary system. It is an excellent inflammation-mediating and anti-allergic herb, very useful for catarrhal conditions, sinusitis, hayfever and asthma.

It is also useful for inflammatory conditions of the bladder and kidneys, including urinary tract infections. It is trophorestorative to the kidneys and where this is needed, long-term use is fine.

Take with caution alongside diuretic medication. Goldenrod is good as an infusion or tincture.

Stachys betonica **wood betony**
Wood betony is a bitter and sedative nervine tonic that has been an important medicinal herb for thousands of years. It is used for mental health problems, especially where someone is very ungrounded, and also where pain is contributing.

Wood betony is helpful with some headaches, specifically those caused by tension, digestive or liver issues as its bitterness will improve weak digestion and gallbladder function. It has also been found to be helpful with pain due to head injuries. Wood betony acts to improve circulation, which will also sometimes help with headaches.

Along with other members of the Lamiaceae family wood betony is recognised as a pain reliever, an inflammation mediator and antioxidant.[113] It also seems to have some action on insulin resistance, lowering a raised blood sugar.

Wood betony should be avoided in pregnancy and breastfeeding, and taken with caution alongside hypotensive and antidiabetic medication.

Symphytum officinale **comfrey leaf**
Comfrey leaf is probably the best vulnerary herb, as its old name of knitbone suggests. It was used internally for arthritis, broken bones and digestive inflammation and ulceration, but since it was determined that it contained liver-damaging pyrrolizidine alkaloids, comfrey is much more likely to be used externally only.

It is still extremely useful externally for any tissue damage, from broken bones to a simple graze of the skin, when made into a poultice or an ointment. It will reduce inflammation and increase collagen deposition,[114] **and result in fast healing, so much so that it should only be used on a clean wound without infection as otherwise an abscess may be formed.**
If used internally it should only be taken short-term, a few weeks at most, and only if there is no liver damage. Comfrey should be avoided in pregnancy or breastfeeding.

Taraxacum officinale **dandelion root and leaf**
Dandelion is a bitter tonic herb that acts as an alterative to improve liver and kidney function. It is an excellent and safe diuretic, and it acts as a cooling and calming liver herb that is useful for those with a hot consti-

tution, hypertension and raised cholesterol levels. Often they also have heartburn and acid reflux, and dandelion will act on digestion to help with this too.

It is a gentle laxative that will move constipation without becoming habit-forming.

Dandelion has been shown to be inflammation-mediating and antioxidant, and is potentially an excellent antidiabetic herb, with many of its individual constituents having blood sugar-lowering and lipid-reducing properties.[115]

The root can be taken as a decoction, roasted or not, the leaves can be eaten or made into an infusion, and both can be made into a tincture.

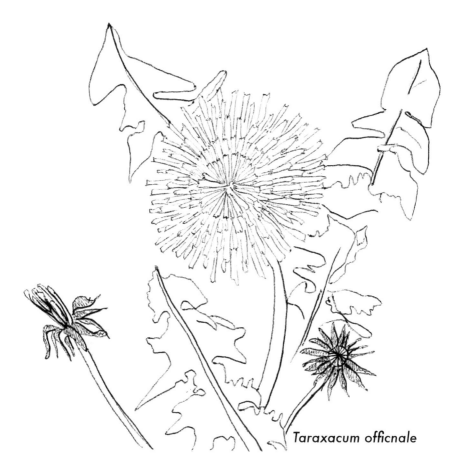

Taraxacum officnale

Thymus spp., *T. vulgaris*, *T. mastichina* **thyme**
Thyme has been recognised as a good antimicrobial, inflammation-mediating and immunomodulatory agent for several thousand years.[116] It is used for cold, stagnant conditions with thick, stuck mucus, and is considered specific for whooping cough[117] as well as all forms of respiratory infections and mucus-forming disorders. It is also a good digestive herb, useful when digestion is sluggish with flatulence.

Thyme is also an excellent tonic and restorative to the nervous system, and it improves memory and concentration and resilience to stress.[118]

As it is also a uterine stimulant it is contraindicated in pregnancy.

Thyme is used as an infusion, tincture or essential oil.

There are many different thymes, all with slightly different profiles but essentially all exhibit these properties.

Tilia europaeus **lime tree or linden flowers**
Linden flower was traditionally used for epilepsy and convulsions as it is a sedative nervine relaxant herb. It is also inflammation-mediating and a cardiac tonic, and it can act as a peripheral vasodilator.

Linden is cooling and calming, and is helpful for any condition of tension, including hypertension, nervous tension, anxiety and palpitations. It will relieve tension headaches and is helpful for insomnia as it is sympatholytic (calming to the sympathetic nervous system).

It makes a lovely infusion, tasting of honey, and mixes well with marshmallow leaf, which makes it less drying.

There are no contraindications for lime flower.

Trametes (Coriolus) versicolor **turkey tail fungus**
This is the most researched medicinal fungus, although most research has been done on the polysaccharide extracts, PSK and PSP. It has been shown to prevent and treat infections and inflammation of the upper respiratory, urinary and digestive tracts; it is also antiviral and has been successfully used for hepatitis.

It is immunomodulating, and is often used to support the immune system during chemotherapy and radiotherapy. It is used to treat and prevent cancer, and it is able to regulate cholesterol and reduce insulin resistance.[119]

Inflammation

Turkey tail is very commonly found in the wild and is easy to identify. It can be decocted and drunk as a tea, or bought as a readymade powder.

Trifolium pratense **red clover**
Red clover is a cooling and moistening alterative with an affinity for the lymphatic system. It is a good inflammation mediator and antioxidant,[120] shows antiangiogenic properties[121] and increases autophagy and apoptosis,[122] making it a useful herb in the treatment of cancer.

It is also a useful herb for the treatment of inflammatory skin conditions.

Red clover should be avoided in pregnancy and breastfeeding. It makes a nice infusion and can also be taken as a tincture.

Trigonella foenum-graecum **fenugreek seed**
Fenugreek is an inflammation-mediating carminative. It has been shown to be antidiabetic, with the ability to reduce blood sugar levels,[123] fatty liver and waist measurement in the obese.[124].

Fenugreek is very helpful in metabolic syndrome, where it can simply be taken as a food.

Ulmus fulva **slippery elm**
Slippery elm contains mucilaginous polysaccharides, which are very soothing and healing to inflamed mucous membranes. It is also an excellent source of prebiotics, which encourage a healthy gut microbiome.

It is useful for all digestive inflammatory conditions, including ulcers, colitis and irritable bowel; and also useful for inflammatory lung conditions such as bronchitis, asthma and pleurisy.

Slippery elm is taken as a powder, which can be mixed in food or drink.

Uncaria tomentosa **cat's claw**
Cat's claw is a South American adaptogen with strong inflammation-mediating action, and has been shown to modulate cytokines, specifically to decrease IL-6 and TNF and increase IL-1.[125,126]

Any condition with lowered immunity or autoimmunity can benefit from cat's claw as it is such a good immune-modulating herb – so this might include chronic fatigue, cancer, rheumatoid arthritis and inflammatory bowel disease. Allergies also benefit from its use.

Cat's claw should be avoided in pregnancy and breastfeeding, and alongside anticoagulant medication. It should be taken with caution alongside hypotensive medication.

Urtica dioica **nettle leaf**
Nettle leaf is a fundamental of Western herbal medicine. It has very many useful properties and is a nutritionally excellent food. Nettle leaf is a trophorestorative for the blood, as it contains minerals, including iron, and chlorophyll.

Nettle leaf also provides support for complex metabolic disorders as it is also an excellent alterative, hypoglycaemic, circulation enhancer and inflammation mediator – examples are allergies, autoimmune disease, metabolic syndrome and inflammatory skin disease. They also have an antihistamine effect.

One study showed that, alongside fish oils and vitamin E, nettle was able to reduce the need for pain medication substantially in osteoarthritis.[127]

Nettle stings are very helpful topically for any sore or arthritic joints, as well as carpal tunnel disease. I have had many people do this and avoid surgery.

Nettle leaf makes a good infusion, and it can be used to make soup, or eaten in the same way as spinach. Nettle leaf can also be taken as a powder or tincture.

There are no contraindications for nettle leaf.

Verbascum thapsus **mullein leaf and flower**
Mullein has been used for many generations as an inflammation-mediating, demulcent, expectorant, antitussive and bronchodilator for respiratory diseases and coughs.[128,129,130]

It acts as an alterative for the lymphatic system, clearing swollen glands and lymphatic congestion. It is excellent for dry coughs, asthma, croup and pleurisy, and can be taken as an infusion or tincture. There are no contraindications.

Verbena officinalis **vervain**
Vervain has a very long tradition of use and was a sacred herb to the Druids, who considered it to be a holy herb. Through medieval times it was

considered a protective herb. It is bitter and cooling, and inflammation-mediating, acting on the liver to calm down over activity and heat, and on the nervous system to relieve anxiety, tension and irritability. It is good for headaches caused by liver heat, and pain, especially when nerve-related.

Vervain is a useful herb for those with chronic fatigue who try too hard, and end up overexerting themselves.

Vervain makes a good infusion, or it can be taken as a tincture or flower essence.

Vervain is a uterine stimulant and should be avoided in pregnancy.

Viola odorata **sweet violet**
Viola tricolor **heartsease**
Sweet violet and heartsease herbs are fairly similar: both are cooling, moistening, inflammation-mediating and alterative, acting on the lymphatic system.

Sweet violet is more appropriate for coughs, colds and bronchial congestion, and is an important aid in the treatment of cancer, with lymphatic infiltration such as breast and lung cancers. Heartsease is more appropriate for inflammatory skin problems.

Both *Violas* make a nice infusion, but can also be taken as a tincture.

Viscum album **mistletoe**
Mistletoe is used today largely for its nervine, antispasmodic, hypotensive and vasodilator actions, which make it a good herb for stress-related high blood pressure, angina and palpitations. It is also helpful for any kind of nervous tension, and for panic attacks.

A fermented preparation of mistletoe is used in the treatment of cancer,[131] and this has been shown to be strongly inflammation-mediating.[132] There is no similar research on unfermented mistletoe products, but they may also have similar effects on inflammation. Mistletoe should be avoided in pregnancy.

Withania somnifera **ashwagandha**
Ashwaganda is an important adaptogen that has been used in Indian traditional medicine (Ayurveda) for many years. It has similar properties to *Panax ginseng*, except for the important difference that it is not stimulating.

Materia Medica

So that makes it very useful as a calming sedative, but strengthening tonic herb that is also helpful for improving the quality of sleep.

It is a good inflammation-mediating and immunomodulatory herb and has been shown to improve neurodegeneration and cognitive impairment where this has been caused by inflammation.[133] It is recognised in India as an excellent male rejuvenative tonic and is used for male infertility.

A review showed that ashwagandha possesses anti-inflammatory, anti-tumor, anti-stress, antioxidant, immunomodulatory, hemopoietic and rejuvenating properties. It also appears to exert a positive influence on the endocrine, cardiopulmonary and central nervous systems.[134]

Ashwaganda is an excellent herb for most chronic inflammatory diseases, although it should be taken with caution by those who are constitutionally hot.

It should be used with caution in pregnancy, and only in the late stages, and should be avoided alongside thyroid medication.

Ashwagandha can be taken as powder or tincture.

Zanthoxylum spp. **prickly ash**
Prickly ash is a warming circulatory stimulant with inflammation-mediating and antimicrobial properties. It is particularly useful in cold, chronic conditions with pain such as fibromyalgia, neuralgia, nerve damage, sinusitis and arthritis as it relieves pain while it improves circulation.

Cold conditions of the digestive system as seen in chronic enteritis also benefit from both its stimulant and antimicrobial actions.

Prickly ash is contraindicated in all hot conditions or constitutions. Small doses of tincture are often enough to get a good result.

Zea mays **corn silk**
The silky strands around the cob of corn make a wonderful tea that is demulcent, inflammation-mediating, cooling and healing to the inflamed and irritated mucous membranes of the genito-urinary system.

If taken in quantity (several litres of the tea in a day, just for a few days) at the first sign of bladder or urethral irritation it can often head off an infection.

Inflammation

Corn silk is best taken as a tea, which is very easy to drink. Ginger can be added to increase the anti-inflammatory effect.

Zingiber officinale **ginger**
Ginger is a warming, stimulating antispasmodic herb acting on the digestive system first and then the whole body. Ginger increases blood circulation, improves digestion and reduces nausea. It reduces platelet aggregation, improving blood flow.

Ginger is excellent for pain relief for pain caused by inflammation, bruising, digestive colic, or dysmenorrhoea,[135] and is possibly one of the most potent inflammation-mediating of herbs, as well as having antioxidant and anticancer action.[136]

Ginger is useful for almost any condition where there is chronic inflammation, but it should be avoided by anyone who is constitutionally hot. Ginger can be used internally as a tea or powder, or externally as a poultice.

Ginger should be used cautiously by anyone taking blood-thinning medication.

Glossary of herb actions

Adaptogen
a non-toxic herb that allows the body to normalise its physiology in
response to stressors, increasing resilience to stress.
Alterative
a herb that can restore proper functioning of the body. Some alteratives
improve the eliminatory functions of the various organs, while others
improve general function.
Analgesic
a herb that reduces pain.
Anti-inflammatory
a herb that mediates the effects of inflammation.
Antispasmodic
a herb that reduces smooth muscle spasms.
Antitussive
a herb that reduces coughing.
Anxiolytic
a herb that reduces anxiety and fear.
Astringent
a herb that dries excess moisture and dampness.
Demulcent
a mucilaginous herb that protects and heals mucous membranes and
other body tissues.
Diaphoretic
a herb that promotes sweating, which can reduce a fever, and also
improve skin elimination.
Diffusive
a herb that breaks up stagnant energy and moves it through the body.
Expectorant
a herb that can loosen and help expel inappropriate or excessive mucus.
$GABA_A$ agonist
a herb that can occupy a $GABA_A$ receptor site in the nervous system,
which induces relaxation and sedation.
Hepatoprotective
a herb that has the ability to protect the liver.
Hypnotic
a herb that promotes sleep.
Immunomodulatory
a herb that can upregulate or down regulate the immune system as
needed, usually an adaptogen.

Nervine
a herb that acts as a tonic for the nervous system, promoting relaxation without sedation, and relieving anxiety and symptoms caused by stress.
Parasympatholytic
is also vagolytic, a herb that is able to improve vagal nerve action and parasympathetic action. It is not the opposite of parasympathomimetic.
Parasympathomimetic
a herb that helps to put the body back into parasympathetic dominance, which is a state of nervous system relaxation.
Phyto-oestrogenic
a herb able to occupy oestrogen receptor sites, which fools the body into thinking it has more oestrogen.
Sedative
a herb that reduce nervous activity.
Sympatholytic
a herb that reduces the physiological results of sympathetic nervous system activity.
Thymoleptic
a herb that lifts the spirits.
Trophorestorative
– also known as tonic herbs – a herb that nourishes, strengthens and restores a body system.
Vulnerary
a herb that promotes wound healing.

Appendix

The major inflammation-mediating herbs and their areas of action

	cir	res	dig	u/k	rep	ms	ns	imm	top
Achillea millefolium	x	x	x	x	x	x		x	x
Aesculus hippocastanum	x								x
Agrimonia eupatoria			x	x		x			
Alchemilla mollis					x				
Allium sativum	x	x	x						x
Angelica archangelica		x	x			x			
Angelica sinensis					x		x	x	
Apium graveolens		x		x		x			
Arctostaphylos uva ursi				x					
Arnica montana	x								x
Asclepias tuberosa	x	x	x						
Berberis vulgaris			x			x			x
Boswellia serrata	x	x	x			x		x	
Calendula officinalis			x		x				x
Cannabis indica/sativa						x	x		
Centella asiatica	x					x	x	x	
Chamaemelum nobile			x						x
Cinnamomum spp.	x	x	x	x	x		x		
Commiphora spp.	x	x	x		x	x			x
Crataegus spp	x						x		
Curcuma longa	x		x	x		x			x
Dioscorea villosa			x		x	x			
Echinacea spp.		x	x	x	x			x	
Euphrasia officinalis		x					x	x	
Filipendula ulmaria			x	x		x			
Foeniculum vulgare			x						

	cir	res	dig	u/k	rep	ms	ns	imm	top
Fucus vesiculosus				x	x	x			x
Ganoderma lucidum	x						x	x	
Glechoma hederacea		x	x	x					
Glycyrrhiza glabra		x	x	x	x			x	x
Harpagophytum procumbens	x		x			x			
Hydrastis canadensis		x	x						x
Hypericum perforatum			x				x		
Hyssopus officinalis		x							
Lavandula spp.		x	x				x		x
Linum usitatissimum		x	x						x
Mahonia aquifolium			x						x
Matricaria recutita		x	x				x		x
Mentha piperita		x	x		x				
Ocimum sanctum	x	x	x	x			x	x	x
Paeonia lactiflora	x				x		x		
Plantago major, P. lanceolata		x	x	x				x	x
Phytolacca american/decandra	x								
Salix spp						x			
Salvia officinalis		x			x		x		x
Salvia rosmarinus	x		x			x	x		
Sambucus nigra		x							x
Scutellaria baicalensis	x	x	x					x	
S. lateriflora			x				x		
Serenoa repens				x	x				
Silybum marianum			x	x					
Smilax glabra				x	x	x			

	cir	res	dig	u/k	rep	ms	ns	imm	top
Solidago virgaurea		x		x	x	x		x	x
Tabebuia impetiginosa		x	x			x			
Tanacetum parthenium			x			x		x	
Thymus vulgaris		x	x						x
Tilia europaea	x	x					x		
Tinospora cordifolia		x	x			x		x	
Ulmus fulva		x	x	x					
Uncaria tomentosa	x	x	x			x		x	
Urtica dioica fol				x		x		x	
Verbascum thapsus		x							
Verbena officinalis				x			x		
Viola odorata		x		x					
V.tricolor	x	x		x					
Withania somnifera				x	x	x	x	x	
Zea mays				x					
Zingiber officinale	x	x	x		x	x		x	

Key:
cir – circulatory / cardiovascular
res – respiratory tract
dig – digestive system including liver
u/k – urinary tract and kidneys
rep – reproductive system
ms – musculoskeletal
ns – nervous system
imm – immune system
top – topical

Notes to the text

Chapter 1, pages 11–18
1. S. Kany et al. Cytokines in inflammatory disease. *Int J Mol. Sci.* 20,23 6008. 28 Nov. 2019.

Chapter 2, pages 19–24
1. R. Jukema et al. Does low-density lipoprotein cholesterol induce inflammation? If so, does it matter? Current insights and future perspectives for novel therapies. *BMC Med* 17, 197 (2019).

Chapter 3, pages 25–48
1. G. Vighi et al. Allergy and the gastrointestinal system. *Clin Exp Immunol*. 153 Suppl 1 (2008): 3–6.
2. L. Galluzzi et al. Autophagy in malignant transformation and cancer progression. *EMBO J* 34,7 (2015): 856–880.
3. P. Kuballa et al. Autophagy and the immune system. *Ann Rev Immunol.* (2012);30: 611–646.
4. L. Shen et al. Dietary PUFAs attenuate NLRP3 inflammasome activation via enhancing macrophage autophagy. *J Lip Res* 58,9 (2017): 1808–1821.
5. J. Bland. The long haul of COVID-19 recovery: immune rejuvenation versus immune support. *IHCAN*, 21 April.
6. N.H. Abdurachman et al. The role of psychological well-being in boosting immune response: an optimal effort for tackling infection. *African J Infect Dis*. 12,1 Suppl 54–61. 7 Mar. 2018.
7. Y. Barak. The immune system and happiness. *Autoimmunity Rev*. 5, 8 (Oct. 2006): 523–527.
8. S. Brod et al. 'As above, so below': examining the interplay between emotion and the immune system. *Immunology* (2014);143(3): 311–318.
9. M. Irwin et al. Partial night sleep deprivation reduces natural killer and cellular immune responses in humans. *FASEB J*. 1996 Apr;10(5):643–653.
10. L.M. Jurkić et al. Biological and therapeutic effects of ortho-silicic acid and some ortho-silicic acid-releasing compounds: new perspectives for therapy. *Nutr Metab (Lond)* 10,2 (2013).
11. Harvard Medical School. Bile acids may help regulate gut immunity and inflammation. *ScienceDaily*. www.sciencedaily.com/releases/2020/01/200103141047.htm, accessed 3/12/20.
12. M. Wammers et al. Reprogramming of pro-inflammatory human macrophages to an anti-inflammatory phenotype by bile acids. *Scientific Rep* 8,1 255. 10 Jan. 2018.

13. Q. Mu et al. Leaky gut as a danger signal for autoimmune diseases. *Front Immunol.* 2017 May 23;8:598.

14. P.D. Cani et al. Metabolic endotoxemia initiates obesity and insulin resistance. *Diabetes.* 2007 Jul;56(7):1761–1772.

15. G.C. Brown. The endotoxin hypothesis of neurodegeneration. *J Neuroinflammation 16*, 180 (2019).

16. C. Franceschi et al. Inflammaging: a new immune–metabolic viewpoint for age-related diseases. *Nat Rev Endocrinol.* 14 (2018): 576–590.

17. N. Jones et al. Fructose reprogrammes glutamine-dependent oxidative metabolism to support LPS-induced inflammation. *Nat Commun 12*, 1209 (2021).

18. L.H. Zhu et al. Constituents from *Apium graveolens* and their anti-inflammatory effects. *J Asian Nat Prod Res.* 2017 Nov;19(11):1079–1086.

19. M. Souissi et al. Antibacterial and anti-inflammatory activities of cardamom (*Elettaria cardamomum*) extracts: potential therapeutic benefits for periodontal infections. *Anaerobe.* 2020 Feb;61:102089.

20. https://www.teknoscienze.com/Contents/Riviste/PDF/AF4_2015_low_31-35.pdf.

21. J.C. Clemente et al. The role of the gut microbiome in systemic inflammatory disease. *BMJ* 2018;360:j5145.

22. S. Alavi et al. Interpersonal gut microbiome variation drives susceptibility and resistance to cholera infection. *Cell.* 181(7) 2020: 1533–1546.

23. J. Sonnenburg & E. Sonnenburg. Vulnerability of the industrialized microbiota. https://science.sciencemag.org/content/366/6464/eaaw9255/tab-pdf.

24. Gut microbiota may influence COVID-19 severity, immune response. *Medscape*, 11 Jan. 2021.

25. S. Lobionda et al. The role of gut microbiota in intestinal inflammation with respect to diet and extrinsic stressors. *Microorganisms* 7,8 271. 19 Aug. 2019.

26. Z. Xin et al. Interplay between gut microbiota and antimicrobial peptides. *Animal Nutrition* 6,4, December 2020: 389–396.

27. M.W. Tabat et al. Acute effects of butyrate on induced hyperpermeability and tight junction protein expression in human colonic tissues. *Biomolecules* 10,5: 766. 14 May 2020.

28. M.H. Mohajeri et al. Relationship between the gut microbiome and brain function. *Nutrition Rev.* 76,7: 481–496. July 2018.

29. D.I. Alesa et al. The role of gut microbiome in the pathogenesis of psoriasis and the therapeutic effects of probiotics. *J Fam Med & Prim Care* 8,11: 3496–3503. 15 Nov. 2019.

30. D. Davani-Davari et al. Prebiotics: definition, types, sources, mechanisms, and clinical applications. *Foods* 8,3: 92. 9 Mar. 2019.

31. I.D. Croall et al. Cognitive deficit and white matter changes in persons with celiac disease: a population-based study. *Gastroenterology* 158,8 (2020): 2112–2122.

32. S. Rosenberg. *Accessing the Healing Power of the Vagus Nerve* (2017).

33. M. Vasefi et al. Diet associated with inflammation and Alzheimer's disease. *J Alzheimers Dis Rep.* 3, 1 (2019): 299–309.

34. E. Schirmer et al. Bisphenols exert detrimental effects on neuronal signaling in mature vertebrate brains. *Commun Biol* 4 (2021): 465.

35. P. Da Luz et al. *Endothelium and Cardiovascular Diseases: Vascular Biology and Clinical Syndromes* (2018).

36. S.R. Gundry, Abstract 10712: Mrna COVID vaccines dramatically increase endothelial inflammatory markers and ACS risk as measured by the PULS cardiac test: a warning. *Circulation* 144 (2021): A10712.

37. R. Kesavan et al. *Gentiana lutea* exerts anti-atherosclerotic effects by preventing endothelial inflammation and smooth muscle cell migration. *Nutr Metab Cardiovasc Dis.* 26, 4 (2016): 293–301.

Chapter 4, pages 49–72.

1. C.J. Murray et al. Global burden of 87 risk factors in 204 countries and territories, 1990–2019: a systematic analysis for the Global Burden of Disease Study 2019. *Lancet* 396, 10258 (2020): 1223–1249.

2. GBD 2017 Diet Collaborators. Health effects of dietary risks in 195 countries, 1990–2017: a systematic analysis for the Global Burden of Disease Study 2017. *Lancet* 393, 10184 (2019): 1958–1972.

3. Dai Haijiang et al. The global burden of disease attributable to high body mass index in 195 countries and territories, 1990–2017: an analysis of the Global Burden of Disease Study. *PLoS Med.* 17, 7 (2020): e1003198.

4. C.A. Daley et al. A review of fatty acid profiles and antioxidant content in grass-fed and grain-fed beef. *Nutr J* 9, 10 (2010).

5. F. Arya et al. Differences in postprandial inflammatory responses to a 'modern' v. traditional meat meal: a preliminary study. *Br J Nutr.* 104, 5 (2010): 724–728.

6. L. Ferrucci et al. Inflammageing: chronic inflammation in ageing, cardiovascular disease, and frailty. *Nat Rev Cardiol.* 15, 9 (2018): 505–522.

7. C. Franceschi et al. Inflammaging: a new immune–metabolic viewpoint for age-related diseases. *Nat Rev Endocrinol.* 14, 10 (2018): 576–590.

8. Ibid.

9. O. Bereshchenko et al. Glucocorticoids, sex hormones, and immunity. *Front Immunol.* 9 (2018): 1332.

10. L. Ferrucci et al. Inflammageing: chronic inflammation in ageing, cardiovascular disease, and frailty. *Nat Rev Cardiol.* 15, 9 (2018): 505–522.

11. M.S. Ellulu et al. Obesity and inflammation: the linking mechanism and the complications. *Arch Med Sci.* 13, 4 (2017): 851–863.

12. C. Franceschi et al. Inflammaging: a new immune–metabolic viewpoint for age-related diseases. *Nat Rev Endocrinol.* 14, 10 (2018): 576–590.

13. J. Pereira et al. The impact of ghrelin in metabolic diseases: an immune perspective. *J Diabetes Res.* (2017): 4527980.

14. G. Pradhan et al. Ghrelin: much more than a hunger hormone. *Curr Opinion Clin Nut & Metabolic Care* 16, 6 (2013): 619–624.

15. M.E. Renna et al. The association between anxiety, traumatic stress, and obsessive-compulsive disorders and chronic inflammation: a systematic review and meta-analysis. *Depress Anxiety* 35, 11 (2018): 1081–1094.

16. M.O. Welcome et al. Stress-induced blood brain barrier disruption: molecular mechanisms and signaling pathways. *Pharmacol Res.* 157 (2020): 104769.

17. S. Dimitrov et al. Inflammation and exercise: inhibition of monocytic intracellular TNF production by acute exercise via β2-adrenergic activation. *Brain Behav Immun* 61 (2017): 60–68.

18. P.M. Preshaw. Detection and diagnosis of periodontal conditions amenable to prevention. *BMC Oral Health* 15, Suppl 1 (2015): S5.

19. V. Sampson. *From Oral Health to Systemic Health: A Dentist's Guide.* Webinar, 2 March 2021.

20. G. Cecoro et al. Periodontitis, low-grade inflammation and systemic health: a scoping review." *Medicina* (Kaunas, Lithuania) 56, 6 (2020): 272. doi:10.3390/medicina56060272.

21. A.N. Gurav. The implication of periodontitis in vascular endothelial dysfunction. *Eur J Clin Invest.* 44, 10 (2014): 1000–1009.

22. M. Paizan et al. Is there an association between periodontitis and hypertension? *Curr Card Rev.* 10, 4 (2014): 355–361.

23. P.M. Preshaw et al. Periodontitis and diabetes: a two-way relationship. *Diabetologia* 55, 1 (2012): 21–31.

24. P. Dahiya et al. Obesity, periodontal and general health: relationship and management. *Indian J Endocr & Metab.* 16, 1 (2012): 88–93.

25. M. Beydoun et al. Clinical and bacterial markers of periodontitis and their association with incident all-cause and Alzheimer's disease dementia in a large national survey. *J Alzheimers Dis* 75, 1 (2020): 157–172.

26. D.V. Parke et al. Chemical-induced inflammation and inflammatory diseases. *Int J Occup Med Environ Health* 9, 3 (1996): 211–217.

27. S. Bondy. Metal toxicity, inflammation and oxidative stress. In S. Bondy & A. Campbell (eds), *Inflammation, Aging, and Oxidative Stress.*

Oxidative Stress in Applied Basic Research and Clinical Practice (2016).

28. R.M. Gardner et al. Mercury induces an unopposed inflammatory response in human peripheral blood mononuclear cells in vitro. *Envir Health Persp.* 117, 12 (2009): 1932–1938.

29. A.O. Summers et al. Mercury released from dental 'silver' fillings provokes an increase in mercury- and antibiotic-resistant bacteria in oral and intestinal floras of primates. *Antimicrob Agents Chemother.* 37, 4 (1993): 825–834.

30. M.Houston. Role of mercury toxicity in hypertension, cardiovascular disease, and stroke. *J Clin Hypertens.* 13 (2011): 621–627.

31. S.-S. Zhou et al. The skin function: a factor of anti-metabolic syndrome. *Diabetol Metab Syndr.* 4, 1 (2012): 15.

32. P. Holmes. *The Energetics of Western Herbs*, 4th ed. (2007): 136.

Chapter 5, pages 73–110

1. L. Ferrucci et al. Inflammaging: chronic inflammation in ageing, cardiovascular disease, and frailty. *Nature Rev. Cardiology* 15, 9 (2018): 505–522.

2. J.A. Bellanti et al. Inflammation and allergic disease: an irrefutable combination. *Allergy and Asth Proc.* 40, 1 (2019): 1–3.

3. J. Sokolove et al. Role of inflammation in the pathogenesis of osteoarthritis: latest findings and interpretations. *Therap Adv in Musculoskeletal Dis.* 5, 2 (2013): 77–94.

4. L. Duan et al. Regulation of inflammation in autoimmune disease. *J Immunol Res.* 2019 (2019): 7403796.

5. M. Rojas et al. Molecular mimicry and autoimmunity. *J Autoimmun.* 95 (2018): 100–123.

6. C. Pinto et al. Role of inflammation and proinflammatory cytokines in cholangiocyte pathophysiology. *Biochim Biophys Acta Mol Basis Dis.* 1864, 4 Pt B (2018): 1270–1278.

7. G. Landskron et al. Chronic inflammation and cytokines in the tumor microenvironment. *J Immunol Res.* 2014 (2014): 149185.

8. L. M. Coussens et al. Inflammation and cancer. *Nature* 420, 6917 (2002): 860–867.

9. P. Libby. Inflammation and cardiovascular disease mechanisms. *Am J Clin Nutr.* 83, 2 (2006): 456S–460S.

10. E. Golia et al. Inflammation and cardiovascular disease: from pathogenesis to therapeutic target. *Curr Atheroscler Rep.* 16, 9 (2014): 435.

11. S.F. Weng et al. Can machine-learning improve cardiovascular risk prediction using routine clinical data? *PLoS One* 12, 4 (2017): e0174944.

12. C. Franceschi et al. Inflammaging: a new immune–metabolic viewpoint for age-related diseases. *Nat Rev Endocrinol.* 14 (2018): 576–590.

13. M. G. Saklayen, The global epidemic of the metabolic syndrome.

Curr Hypertension Reps. 20, 2 (2018): 12.

14. N. Stefan et al. Causes, characteristics, and consequences of metabolically unhealthy normal weight in humans. *Cell Metabol.* 26 (2017): 292–300.

15. A. Lopez-Candales et al. Linking chronic inflammation with cardiovascular disease: from normal aging to the metabolic syndrome. *J Nat & Sci.* 3, 4 (2017): e341.

16. C. Thaiss et al. Hyperglycemia drives intestinal barrier dysfunction and risk for enteric infection. *Science* 359 (2018): 1376–1383.

17. W.H. Tang. Gut microbiota in cardiovascular health and disease. *Circ Res.* 120 (2017): 1183–1196.

18. P.M. Preshaw et al. Periodontitis and diabetes. *Br Dent J* 227, 7 (2019): 577–584.

19. M. O'Hearn et al. Coronavirus disease 2019 hospitalizations attributable to cardiometabolic conditions in the United States: a comparative risk assessment analysis. *J Am Heart Ass.* 10 (2021): e019259.

20. T.T. Nguyen et al. Type 3 diabetes and its role implications in Alzheimer's disease. *Int J Mol Sci.* 21, 9 (2020), 3165.

21. N. Namazi et al. The effect of hydro alcoholic nettle (*Urtica dioica*) extracts on insulin sensitivity and some inflammatory indicators in patients with type 2 diabetes: a randomized double-blind control trial. *Pak J Biol Sci.* 14, 15 (2011): 775–779.

22. N. Suksomboon et al. Meta-analysis of the effect of herbal supplement on glycemic control in type 2 diabetes. *J Ethnopharmacol.* 137, 3 (2011): 1328–1333.

23. M. Rohr. Inflammatory diseases of the gut. *J Medic Food* 21, 2 (2018): 113–126.

24. B. Moldoveanu et al. Inflammatory mechanisms in the lung. *J Inflamm Res.* 2 (2009): 1–11.

25. D.I. Alesa et al. The role of gut microbiome in the pathogenesis of psoriasis and the therapeutic effects of probiotics. *J Fam Med & Prim Care* 8, 11 (2019): 3496–3503.

26. L. Guzman-Martinez et al. Neuroinflammation as a common feature of neurodegenerative disorders. *Front Pharmacol.* 10 (2019): 1008.

27. J.A. Nicoll et al. Persistent neuropathological effects 14 years following amyloid-β immunization in Alzheimer's disease. *Brain* 142, 7 (2019): 2113–2126.

28. E.M. Borsom et al. Do the bugs in your gut eat your memories? Relationship between gut microbiota and Alzheimer's disease. *Brain Sci.* 10, 11 (2020): 814.

29. G.C. Brown. The endotoxin hypothesis of neurodegeneration. *J Neuroinflammation* 16, 1 (2019): 180.

30. M. Marizzoni et al. Short-chain fatty acids and lipopolysaccharide as

mediators between gut dysbiosis and amyloid pathology in Alzheimer's disease. *J Alzheimers Dis.* 78, 2 (2020): 683–697.

31. M. Beydoun et al. Clinical and bacterial markers of periodontitis and their association with incident all-cause and Alzheimer's disease dementia in a large national survey. *J Alzheimers Dis.* 75, 1 (2020): 157–172.

32. S.R. Irani et al. The neuroinflammation collection: a vision for expanding neuro-immune crosstalk in *Brain*. *Brain* 144, 7 (2021): e59.

33. D. Bredesen. *The End of Alzheimers* (2017).

34. K. Dhana et al. MIND diet, common brain pathologies, and cognition in community-dwelling older adults. *J Alzheimers Dis.* 83, 2 (2021): 683–692.

35. https://www.psychiatrictimes.com/view/introduction-inflammation-connection.

36. L. Chieh-Hsin et al. The role of inflammation in depression and fatigue. *Front Immunol.* 10 (2019): 1696.

37. J. Firth et al. Food and mood: how do diet and nutrition affect mental wellbeing? *BMJ* 2020;369:m2382.

38. L. Ginaldi et al. Osteoporosis, inflammation and ageing. *Immun Ageing* 2 (2005): 14.

39. A.S. Nazrun et al. The anti-inflammatory role of Vitamin E in prevention of osteoporosis. *Adv Pharma Sci.* 2012 (2012): 142702.

Chapter 6, pages 111–132

1. J. Firth et al. Food and mood: how do diet and nutrition affect mental wellbeing? *BMJ* 2020;369:m2382.

2. N. Jones et al. Fructose reprogrammes glutamine-dependent oxidative metabolism to support LPS-induced inflammation. *Nat Commun.* 12 (2021): 1209.

3. A.Kumthekar et al. Obesity and psoriatic arthritis: a narrative review. *Rheumatol & Therapy* 7, 3 (2020): 447–456.

4. M. Rojas et al. Molecular mimicry and autoimmunity. *J Autoimmun.* 95 (2018): 100–123.

5. M. Nanayakkara et al. P31–43, an undigested gliadin peptide, mimics and enhances the innate immune response to viruses and interferes with endocytic trafficking: a role in celiac disease. *Sci Rep.* 8 (2018): 10821.

6. A. Samsel et al. Glyphosate, pathways to modern diseases II: celiac sprue and gluten intolerance. *Interdiscip Toxicol.* 6, 4 (2013): 159–184.

7. Y. Zhu et al. Dietary total fat, fatty acids intake, and risk of cardiovascular disease: a dose-response meta-analysis of cohort studies. *Lipids in Health & Dis.* 18, 1 (2019), 91. doi:10.1186/s12944-019-1035-2.

8. A. Malhotra et al. Saturated fat does not clog the arteries: coronary heart disease is a chronic inflammatory condition, the risk of which can

be effectively reduced from healthy lifestyle interventions. *Br J Sports Med.* 51 (2017): 1111–1112.

9. R.J. de Souza et al. Intake of saturated and trans unsaturated fatty acids and risk of all-cause mortality, cardiovascular disease, and type 2 diabetes: systematic review and meta-analysis of observational studies. *BMJ* 2015;351:h3978.

10. https://theconsciouslife.com/omega-3-6-9-ratio-cooking-oils.htm.

11. E. Hsu et al. Anti-inflammatory and antioxidant effects of sesame oil on atherosclerosis: a descriptive literature review. *Cureus* 9, 7 (2017): e1438.

12. M. Marklund et al. Biomarkers of dietary omega-6 fatty acids and incident cardiovascular disease and mortality: an individual-level pooled analysis of 30 cohort studies. *Circulation* 139 (2019): 21.

13. S. Okparanta et al. Assessment of rancidity and other physicochemical properties of edible oils (mustard and corn oils) stored at room temperature. *J Food & Nutr Sci.* 6, 3 (2018): 70–75.

14. S. Jew et al. Evolution of the human diet: linking our ancestral diet to modern functional foods as a means of chronic disease prevention. *J Medic Food* 12, 5 (2009): 925–934.

15. ibid.

16. S. Myhill & C. Robinson. *The PK Cookbook* (2017).

17. http://www.christineherbert.co.uk/articles/histamine/.

18. O. Comas-Basté et al. Histamine intolerance: the current state of the art. *Biomolecules* 10, 8 (2020): 1181. doi:10.3390/biom10081181.

19. J. Aparecida da Silva Pereira et al. The impact of ghrelin in metabolic diseases: an immune perspective. *J Diabetes Res.* 2017 (2017): 4527980.

20. M.C. Phillips. Fasting as a therapy in neurological disease. *Nutrients* 11,10 (Oct. 2019): 2501.

21. C. Franceschi et al. Inflammaging: a new immune–metabolic viewpoint for age-related diseases. *Nat Rev Endocrinol.* 14 (2018): 576–590.

22. ibid.

23. M.A-Islam E. Faris et al. Ramadan intermittent fasting and immunity: an important topic in the era of COVID-19. *Ann Thorac Med.* 15, 3 (2020): 125–133.

Chapter 7, pages 133–142

1. R. Farré et al. Intestinal permeability, inflammation and the role of nutrients. *Nutrients* 12, 4 (2020): 1185.

2. Zhiyi Huang et al. Role of vitamin A in the immune system. *J Clin Med.* 7, 9 (2018): 258.

3. R. Reifen. Vitamin A as an anti-inflammatory agent. *Proc Nutr Soc.* 61, 3 (2002): 397–400.

4. K. Poudel-Tandukar et al. Dietary B vitamins and serum C-reactive protein in persons with Human Immunodeficiency Virus infection: the Positive Living with HIV (POLH) study. *Food Nutr Bull.* 37, 4 (2016): 517–528.

5. M. Markišić et al. The impact of homocysteine, vitamin B12, and vitamin D levels on functional outcome after first-ever ischaemic stroke. *BioMed Res Int.* 2017 (2017): 5489057.

6. S.C. Huang et al. Vitamin B6 supplementation improves pro-inflammatory responses in patients with rheumatoid arthritis. *Eur J Clin Nutr.* 64 (2010): 1007–1013.

7. E.P. Chiang et al. Inflammation causes tissue-specific depletion of vitamin B6. *Arthritis Res Ther.* 7 (2005): R1254.

8. A.C. Carr et al. Vitamin C and immune function. *Nutrients* 9, 11 (2017): 1211.

9. M.S. Ellulu et al. Effect of vitamin C on inflammation and metabolic markers in hypertensive and/or diabetic obese adults: a randomized controlled trial. *Drug Design, Devel & Ther.* 9 (2015): 3405–3412.

10. M.A. Moser et al. Vitamin C and heart health: a review based on findings from epidemiologic studies. *Intern J Mol Sci.* 17, 8 (2016): 1328.

11. J.M. Pullar et al. The roles of vitamin C in skin health. *Nutrients* 9, 8 (2017): 866.

12. J. Fletcher et al. The role of vitamin D in iInflammatory bowel disease: mechanism to management. *Nutrients* 11, 5 (2019): 1019.

13. https://www.webmed.com/cancer/news/20111004/low-vitamin-d-levels-linked-to-advanced-cancers#1.

14. E.K. Weir et al. Does vitamin D deficiency increase the severity of COVID-19? *Clin Med* (London, England) 20, 4 (2020): e107–e108.

15. R. Farré et al. Intestinal permeability, inflammation and the role of nutrients. *Nutrients* 12, 4 (2020): 1185.

16. M. Markišić et al. The impact of homocysteine, vitamin B12, and vitamin D levels on functional outcome after first-ever ischaemic stroke. *BioMed Res Int.* 2017 (2017): 5489057.

17. T. Passeron et al. Sunscreen protection and vitamin D status. *Br J Dermatol.* 181, 5 (2019): 916–931.

18. A.R. Webb et al. Meeting vitamin D requirements in white Caucasians at UK latitudes: providing a choice. *Nutrients* 10, 4 (2018): 497.

19. M.F. Holick et al. Evaluation, treatment, and prevention of vitamin D deficiency: an Endocrine Society Clinical Practice Guideline. *J Clin Endocrinol Metab.* 96, 7 (2011): 1911–1930.

20. O. Asbaghi et al. The effect of vitamin E supplementation on selected inflammatory biomarkers in adults: a systematic review and meta-analysis of randomized clinical trials. *Sci Rep.* 10 (2020): 17234.

21. A.S. Nazrun et al. The anti-inflammatory role of vitamin E in

Notes

prevention of osteoporosis. *Adv Pharm Sci.* 2012 (2012): 142702.

22. F.H. Nielsen. Magnesium deficiency and increased inflammation: current perspectives. *J Inflamm Res.* 11 (2018): 25–34.

23. J.J. Di Nicolantonio et al. Subclinical magnesium deficiency: a principal driver of cardiovascular disease and a public health crisis. *Open Heart* 5, 1 (2018): e000668.

24. E. Serefko et al. Magnesium in depression. *Pharmacol Rep.* 65, 3 (2013): 547–554.

25. F.H. Nielsen. Magnesium deficiency and increased inflammation: current perspectives. *J Inflamm Res.* 11 (2018): 25–34.

26. M. Mazidi et al. Effect of magnesium supplements on serum C-reactive protein: a systematic review and meta-analysis. *Arch Med Sci.* 14, 4 (2018): 707–716.

27. A.S. Prasad. Zinc: An antioxidant and anti-inflammatory agent: role of zinc in degenerative disorders of aging. *J Trace Elem Med Biol.* 28, 4 (2014): 364–371.

28. N.Z. Gammoh et al. Zinc in infection and inflammation. *Nutrients* 9, 6 (2017): 624.

29. Z. Huang et al. The role of selenium in inflammation and immunity: from molecular mechanisms to therapeutic opportunities. *Antioxid Redox Signal.* 16, 7 (2012): 705–743.

30. L.H. Duntas et al. Selenium and inflammation – potential use and future perspectives. *US Endocrinol.* 11, 2 (2015): 97–102.

31. P.R. Souza et al. Enriched marine oil supplements increase peripheral blood specialized pro-resolving mediators concentrations and reprogram host immune responses – a randomized double-blind placebo-controlled study. *Circ Res.* 126, 1 (2020): 75–90.

32. P.E. Miller et al. Long-chain omega-3 fatty acids eicosapentaenoic acid and docosahexaenoic acid and blood pressure: a meta-analysis of randomized controlled trials. *Am J Hypertens.* 27, 7 (2014): 885–896.

33. J.N. Din et al. Effect of ω-3 fatty acid supplementation on endothelial function, endogenous fibrinolysis and platelet activation in male cigarette smokers. *Heart* 99, 3 (2013): 168–174.

34. U. Akbar et al. Omega-3 fatty acids in rheumatic diseases. *J Clin Rheumatol.* 23, 6 (S2017): 330–339.

35. D.M. Djalilova et al. Impact of yoga on inflammatory biomarkers: a systematic review. *Biol Res Nurs.* 21, 2 (2019): 198–209.

36. I. Buric et al. What is the molecular signature of mind–body interventions? A systematic review of gene expression changes induced by meditation and related practices. *Front Immunol.* 16, 8 (2017): 670.

37. J.D. Cresswell et al. Alterations in resting-state functional connectivity link mindfulness meditation with reduced interleukin-6: a randomised controlled trial *Biol Psychiatry* 80, 1 (2016): 53–61.

38. P.L. Gerbarg et al. The effect of breathing, movement, and meditation on psychological and physical symptoms and inflammatory biomarkers in Inflammatory Bowel Disease: a randomized controlled trial. *Inflamm Bowel Diseases* 21, 12 (2015): 2886–2896.

39. J.A. Woods et al. Exercise, inflammation and aging. *Aging & Disease* 3, 1 (2012): 130–140.

40. G.I. Lancaster et al. The immunomodulating role of exercise in metabolic disease. *Trends Immunol.* 35, 6 (2014): 262–269.

41. I. Bjarnason et al. Intestinal permeability in the pathogenesis of NSAID-induced enteropathy. *J Gastroenterol.* 44 Suppl 19 (2009): 23–29.

42. A.P. Bhatt et al. Nonsteroidal anti-inflammatory drug-induced leaky gut modeled using polarized monolayers of primary human intestinal epithelial cells. *ACS Infect Dis.* 4, 1 (2018): 46–52.

43. E. Utzeri et al. Role of non-steroidal anti-inflammatory drugs on intestinal permeability and nonalcoholic fatty liver disease. *World J Gastroenterol.* 23, 22 (2017): 3954–3963.

44. Z. Varga et al. Cardiovascular risk of nonsteroidal anti-inflammatory drugs: an under-recognized public health issue. *Cureus* 9, 4 (2017): e1144.

45. A.M. Schjerning et al. Cardiovascular effects and safety of (non-aspirin) NSAIDs. *Nat Rev Cardiol.* 17 (2020): 574–584.

46. G. Lucas et al. Pathophysiological aspects of nephropathy caused by non-steroidal anti-inflammatory drugs. *Jornal brasileiro de nefrologia* 41, 1 (2019): 124–130.

47. A.R. Cameron et al. Anti-inflammatory effects of metformin irrespective of diabetes status. *Circ Research.* 119 (2016): 652–665.

Chapter 8, pages 143–152
1. D. Winston. *Adaptogens: Herbs for Strength, Stamina, and Stress Relief* (2019).

2. S. Sontakke et al. Open, randomized, controlled clinical trial of *Boswellia serrata* extract as compared to valdecoxib in osteoarthritis of knee. *Indian J Pharmacol.* 39, 1 (2007): 27–29.

3. T. Newmark & P. Schulick, Paul (2000) *Beyond Aspirin: Nature's Answer to Arthritis, Cancer & Alzheimer's Disease* (2000).

4. K. Spelman et al. Modulation of cytokine expression by traditional medicines: a review of herbal immunomodulators. *Altern Med Rev.* 11, 2 (2006): 128–150.

Chapter 9, pages 153–207
1. J. Stansbury. *Herbal Formularies for Health Professionals*, vol. 2: *Circulation and Respiration* (2018).

2. D. Ivanova et al. *Agrimonia eupatoria* tea consumption in relation to markers of inflammation, oxidative status and lipid metabolism in

healthy subjects. *Arch Physiol Biochem.* 119, 1 (2013): 32–37.

3. M. Wood. *The Earthwise Herbal,* vol. 1: *A Complete Guide to Old World Medicinal Plants* (2008).

4. D.S. Butt et al. Garlic: nature's protection against physiological threats. *Crit Rev Food Sci Nutr.* 49, 6 (2009): 538–551.

5. Md S. Hossain et al. *Andrographis paniculata* (Burm. f.) Wall. ex Nees: a review of ethnobotany, phytochemistry, and pharmacology. *ScientificWorldJournal* 2014 (2014): 274905.

6. A. Stableford. *The Handbook of Constitutional and Energetic Herbal Medicine* (2020).

7. ibid.

8. M. Wood. *The Earthwise Herbal,* vol. 1: *A Complete Guide to Old World Medicinal Plants* (2008). 9. L.H. Zhu et al. Constituents from *Apium graveolens* and their anti-inflammatory effects. *J Asian Nat Prod Res.* 19, 11 (2017): 1079–1086.

10. W. Kooti et al. A review of the antioxidant activity of celery (*Apium graveolens* L). *J Evid Based Complement Alternat Med.* 22, 4 (2017): 1029–1034.

11. A. Stableford. *The Handbook of Constitutional and Energetic Herbal Medicine* (2020).

12. C. Herz et al. Evaluation of an aqueous extract from horseradish root (*Armoracia rusticana* radix) against lipopolysaccharide-induced cellular inflammation reaction. *J Evid Based Complement Alternat Med.* (2017): 1950692.

13. R.F. Weiss. *Weiss's Herbal Medicine* (1988).

14. M. Wood. *The Earthwise Herbal,* vol. 1: *A Complete Guide to Old World Medicinal Plants* (2008).

15. H. Ekiert et al. Significance of *Artemisia vulgaris* L. (common mugwort) in the history of medicine and its possible contemporary applications substantiated by phytochemical and pharmacological studies. *Molecules* (Basel, Switzerland) 25, 19 (2020): 4415.

16. A. Stableford. *The Handbook of Constitutional and Energetic Herbal Medicine* (2020).

17. R. Singla et al. Shatavari *Asparagus racemosus*: a review on its cultivation, morphology, phytochemical and pharmacological importance. *Int J Pharma Sci Res.* 5, 3 (2014): 742–757.

18. Y. Zheng et al. A review of the pharmacological action of astragalus polysaccharide. *Front Pharmacol.* 11 (2020): 349.

19. P. Holmes. *The Energetics of Western Herbs* (2006).

20. J. Bruton-Seal & M. Seal. *Wayside Medicine* (2017).

21. X. Feng et al. Berberine in cardiovascular and metabolic diseases: from mechanisms to therapeutics. *Theranostics* 9, 7 (2019): 1923–1951.

22. M. Wood. *The Earthwise Herbal,* vol. 1: *A Complete Guide to Old World*

Medicinal Plants (2008).

23. N.K. Roy et al. An update on pharmacological potential of boswellic acids against chronic diseases. *Int J Mol Sci.* 20, 17 (2019): 4101.

24. M.Z. Siddiqui. *Boswellia serrata*, a potential antiinflammatory agent: an overview. *Indian J Pharma Sci.* 73, 3 (2011): 255–261.

25. S. Sontakke et al. Open, randomized, controlled clinical trial of *Boswellia serrata* extract as compared to valdecoxib in osteoarthritis of knee. *Indian J Pharmacol.* 39, 1 (2007): 27–29.

26. A. McIntyre & M. Boudin. *Dispensing with Tradition: A Practitioner's Guide to Using Indian and Western Herbs the Ayurvedic Way* (2012).

27. S. Atalay et al. Antioxidative and anti-inflammatory properties of cannabidiol. *Antioxidants* (Basel, Switzerland) 9, 1 (2019): 21.

28. H. Khodadadi et al. Cannabidiol ameliorates cognitive function via regulation of IL-33 and TREM2 upregulation in a murine model of Alzheimer's disease. *J Alzheimers Dis* 80, 3 (2021): 973–977.

29. A. Stableford. *The Handbook of Constitutional and Energetic Herbal Medicine* (2020).

30. G. Paun et al. Chemical and bioactivity evaluation of *Eryngium planum* and *Cnicus benedictus* polyphenolic-rich extracts. *BioMed Res Int.* 2019 (2019): 3692605.

31. M. Wood. *The Earthwise Herbal*, vol. 1: *A Complete Guide to Old World Medicinal Plants* (2008).

32. A. Stableford. *The Handbook of Constitutional and Energetic Herbal Medicine* (2020).

33. B. Sun et al. Therapeutic potential of *Centella asiatica* and its triterpenes: a review. *Front Pharmacol.* 11 (2020): 1373.

34. M. Wood. *The Earthwise Herbal*, vol. 1: *A Complete Guide to Old World Medicinal Plants* (2008).

35. J. Stansbury. *Herbal Formularies for Health Professionals*, vol. 1: *Digestion and Elimination* (2018).

36. J. Stansbury. *Herbal Formularies for Health Professionals*, vol. 4: *Neurology, Psychiatry, and Pain Management* (2020).

37. P. Dhanapakiam et al. The cholesterol lowering property of coriander seeds (*Coriandrum sativum*): mechanism of action. *J Environ Bio.* 29, 1 (2008): 53–56.

38. Q. Jabeen et al. Coriander fruit exhibits gut modulatory, blood pressure lowering and diuretic activities. *J Ethnopharmacol.* 122, 1 (2009): 123–130.

39. Y. Zhang et al. A novel analgesic isolated from a traditional Chinese medicine. *Curr Biol.* 24, 2 (2014): 117–123.

40. A. Sahebkar et al. Lipid-lowering activity of artichoke extracts: a systematic review and meta-analysis. *Crit Rev Food Sci Nutr.* 58, 15 (2018): 2549–2556.

Notes   223

41. A. Matthias et al. Echinacea in health – risks and benefits. In R. Watson & V. Preedy (eds), *Botanical Medicine in Clinical Practice* (2008).

42. M. Souissi et al. Antibacterial and anti-inflammatory activities of cardamom (*Elettaria cardamomum*) extracts: potential therapeutic benefits for periodontal infections. *Anaerobe* 61 (2020): 102089.

43. M. Davydov et al. *Eleutherococcus senticosus* (Rupr. & Maxim.) Maxim. (Araliaceae) as an adaptogen: a closer look. *J Ethnopharmacol.* 72, 3 (2000): 345–393.

44. S. Colegate et al. Potentially toxic pyrrolizidine alkaloids in *Eupatorium perfoliatum* and three related species. Implications for herbal use as boneset. *Phytochemical Anal.* 29 (2018): 10.1002/pca.2775.

45. Y. Liu et al. Protective effects of *Euphrasia officinalis* extract against ultraviolet B-induced photoaging in normal human dermal fibroblasts. *Int J Mol Sci.* 19, 11 (2018): 3327.

46. H.S. Lee et al. *Foeniculum vulgare* Mill. protects against lipopolysaccharide-induced acute lung injury in mice through ERK-dependent NF-κB activation. *Korean J Physiol Pharmacol.* 19, 2 (2015): 183–189.

47. T. Ilina et al. Phytochemical profiles and in vitro immunomodulatory activity of ethanolic extracts from *Galium aparine* L. *Plants* (Basel, Switzerland) 8, 12 (2019): 541.

48. Z. Cai et al. Anti-inflammatory activities of *Ganoderma lucidum* (Lingzhi) and San-Miao-San supplements in MRL/lpr mice for the treatment of systemic lupus erythematosus. *Chin Med.* 11 (2016): 23.

49. T. Cafaro et al. Anti-apoptotic and anti-inflammatory activity of *Gentiana lutea* root extract. *Adv Trad Med.* 20, 4 (2020): 619–630.

50. R. Kesavan et al. *Gentiana lutea* exerts anti-atherosclerotic effects by preventing endothelial inflammation and smooth muscle cell migration. *Nutr Metab Cardiovasc Dis.* 26, 4 (2016): 293–301.

51. S. Kaur et al. Anti-inflammatory effects of *Ginkgo* biloba extract against trimethyltin-induced hippocampal neuronal injury. *Inflammopharmacology* 26, 1 (2018): 87–104.

52. T. Zhu et al. Evaluation of the anti-inflammatory properties of the active constituents in *Ginkgo biloba* for the treatment of pulmonary diseases. *Food Funct.* 10 (2019): 2209–2220.

53. B. Gargouri et al. Anti-neuroinflammatory effects of *Ginkgo biloba* extract EGb761 in LPS-activated primary microglial cells. *Phytomedicine* 44 (2018): 45–55.

54. P. Holmes. *The Energetics of Western Herbs* (2007).

55. S. Weinmann et al. Effects of *Ginkgo biloba* in dementia: systematic review and meta-analysis. *BMC Geriatr.* 10 (2010): 14.

56. S.T. Chou et al. Phytochemical profile of hot water extract of *Glechoma hederacea* and its antioxidant, and anti-inflammatory activities.

Inflammation

Life Sci. 231 (2019): 116519.

57. G. Hetland et al. Antitumor, anti-inflammatory and antiallergic effects of *Agaricus blazei* mushroom extract and the related medicinal basidiomycetes mushrooms, *Hericium erinaceus* and *Grifola frondosa*: a review of preclinical and clinical studies. *Nutrients* 12, 5 (2020): 1339.

58. C. Xiao et al. Hypoglycemic effects of *Grifola frondosa* (Maitake) polysaccharides F2 and F3 through improvement of insulin resistance in diabetic rats. *Food Funct.* 6, 11 (2015): 3567–3575.

59. A. McIntyre & M. Boudin. *Dispensing with Tradition: A Practitioner's Guide to Using Indian and Western Herbs the Ayurvedic Way* (2012).

60. L.Y. Zuñiga et al. Effect of *Gymnema sylvestre* administration on metabolic syndrome, insulin sensitivity, and insulin secretion. *J Med Food* 20, 8 (2017): 750–754.

61. A. McIntyre & M. Boudin. *Dispensing with Tradition: A Practitioner's Guide to Using Indian and Western Herbs the Ayurvedic Way* (2012).

62. S. Nandy et al. Indian sarsaparilla (*Hemidesmus indicus*): recent progress in research on ethnobotany, phytochemistry and pharmacology. *J Ethnopharmacol.* 254 (2020): 112609.

63. M. Wood. *The Earthwise Herbal*, vol. 1: *A Complete Guide to Old World Medicinal Plants* (2008).

64. A. McIntyre & M. Boudin. *Dispensing with Tradition: A Practitioner's Guide to Using Indian and Western Herbs the Ayurvedic Way* (2012).

65. S.K. Mandal et al. Goldenseal (*Hydrastis canadensis* L.) and its active constituents: a critical review of their efficacy and toxicological issues. *Pharmacol Res.* 160 (2020): 105085.

66. M. Wood. *The Earthwise Herbal*, vol. 1: *A Complete Guide to Old World Medicinal Plants* (2008).

67. K.V. Ho et al. Black walnut (*Juglans nigra*) extracts inhibit proinflammatory cytokine production from lipopolysaccharide-stimulated human promonocytic cell line U-937. *Front Pharmacol.* 10 (2019): 1059.

68. B. Sadowska et al. The immunomodulatory potential of *Leonurus cardiaca* extract in relation to endothelial cells and platelets. *Innate Immun.* 23, 3 (2017): 285–295.

69. A. McIntyre & M. Boudin. *Dispensing with Tradition: A Practitioner's Guide to Using Indian and Western Herbs the Ayurvedic Way* (2012).

70. M. Wood. *The Earthwise Herbal*, vol. 1: *A Complete Guide to Old World Medicinal Plants* (2008).

71. A. Aziz et al. (2014). In vitro anti-inflammatory activity of *Lycopus europaeus* Linn. *Int J Pharma Sci.* 4 (2014): 689–691.

72. A.M. Beer et al. *Lycopus europaeus* (Gypsywort): effects on the thyroidal parameters and symptoms associated with thyroid function. *Phytomedicine* 15, 1–2 (2008): 16–22.

Notes

73. M. Moore. *Medicinal Plants of the Pacific West* (2001).

74. A. Andreicut et al. Anti-inflammatory and antioxidant effects of *Mahonia aquifolium* leaves and bark extracts. *Farmacia* 66, 1 (2018): 49.

75. M. Aćimović et al. *Marrubium vulgare* L.: a phytochemical and pharmacological overview. *Molecules* 25, 12 (2020): 2898.

76. J.K. Srivastava et al. Chamomile, a novel and selective COX-2 inhibitor with anti-inflammatory activity. *Life Sci.* 85, 19–20 (2009): 663–669.

77. M. Wood. *The Earthwise Herbal*, vol. 1: *A Complete Guide to Old World Medicinal Plants* (2008).

78. K. Świąder et al. The therapeutic properties of Lemon balm (*Melissa officinalis* L.): reviewing novel findings and medical indications. *J App Bot & Food Quality* 92 (2019): 327–335.

79. Y. Li et al. In vitro antiviral, anti-inflammatory, and antioxidant activities of the ethanol extract of *Mentha piperita* L. *Food Sci Biotech.* 26, 6 (2017): 1675–1683.

80. M.M. Cohen. Tulsi – *Ocimum sanctum*: a herb for all reasons. *J Ayurveda & Integ Med.* 5, 4 (2014): 251–259.

81. S. Kang et al. Ginseng, the 'immunity boost': the effects of *Panax ginseng* on immune system. *J Ginseng Res.* 36, 4 (2012): 354–368.

82. A. Shojaii et al. Review of pharmacological properties and chemical constituents of *Pimpinella anisum*. *ISRN Pharmaceutics* 2012 (2012): 510795.

83. M.E. Embuscado. Vanilla, in Encyclopedia of Food Chemistry (2019).

84. I. Türel et al. Hepatoprotective and anti-inflammatory activities of *Plantago major* L. *Indian J Pharmacol.* 41, 3 (2009): 120–124.

85. P. Fan et al. Anti-inflammatory activity of the invasive neophyte *Polygonum cuspidatum* Sieb. and Zucc. (Polygonaceae) and the chemical comparison of the invasive and native varieties with regard to resveratrol. *J Trad Comp Med.* 3, 3 (2013): 182–187.

86. S.H. Buhner. *Healing Lyme Disease Coinfections* (2013).

87. S.J. Wang et al. *Prunella vulgaris*: a comprehensive review of chemical constituents, pharmacological effects and clinical applications. *Curr Pharm Des.* 25, 3 (2019): 359–369.

88. W.L. Pu et al. Anti-inflammatory effects of *Rhodiola rosea* L.: a review. *Biomed Pharmacother.* 121 (2020): 109552.

89. Y. Lee et al. Anti-inflammatory and neuroprotective effects of constituents isolated from *Rhodiola rosea*. *Evid Based Complement Alternat Med.* 2013 (2013): 514049.

90. Y. Lekomtseva et al. *Rhodiola rosea* in subjects with prolonged or chronic fatigue symptoms: results of an open-label clinical trial. *Complement Med Res.* 24, 1 (2017): 46–52.

91. J. Gruenwald et al. *Rosa canina* – Rose hip pharmacological ingredients and molecular mechanics counteracting osteoarthritis – A

Inflammation

systematic review. *Phytomedicine* 60 (2019): 152958.

92. M. Wood. *The Earthwise Herbal*, vol. 1: *A Complete Guide to Old World Medicinal Plants* (2008).

93. T. Eom et al. In vitro antioxidant, antiinflammation, and anticancer activities and anthraquinone content from *Rumex crispus* root extract and fractions. *Antioxidants* (Basel). 9, 8 (2020): 726.

94. B.-Q. Wang. *Salvia miltiorrhiza*: chemical and pharmacological review of a medicinal plant. *J Med Plants Res.* 4, 25 (2010): 2813–2820.

95. Z. Yin et al. *Salvia miltiorrhiza* in anti-diabetic angiopathy. *Curr Mol Pharmacol.* 14, 6 (2021): 960–974.

96. M. Wood. *The Earthwise Herbal*, vol. 1: *A Complete Guide to Old World Medicinal Plants* (2008).

97. A.L. Lopresti. *Salvia* (sage): a review of its potential cognitive-enhancing and protective effects. *Drugs in R&D* 17, 1 (2017): 53–64.

98. A. McIntyre & M. Boudin. *Dispensing with Tradition: A Practitioner's Guide to Using Indian and Western Herbs the Ayurvedic Way* (2012).

99. J.R. de Oliveira et al. *Rosmarinus officinalis* L. (rosemary) as therapeutic and prophylactic agent. *J Biomed Sci.* 26, 1 (2019): 5.

100. M. Nazari et al. Anti-inflammation effects of *Rosmarinus officinalis* extract against Covid19 virus (in silico study). *J Bioequiv & Bioavailab.* 5, 2 (2021).

101. M. Wood. *The Earthwise Herbal*, vol. 1: *A Complete Guide to Old World Medicinal Plants* (2008).

102. J. Zielińska-Wasielica et al. Elderberry (*Sambucus nigra* L.) fruit extract alleviates oxidative stress, insulin resistance, and inflammation in hypertrophied 3T3-L1 adipocytes and activated RAW 264.7 macrophages. *Foods* 8, 8 (2019): 326.

103. A. Nowak et al. Potential of *Schisandra chinensis* (Turcz.) Baill. in human health and nutrition: a review of current knowledge and therapeutic perspectives. *Nutrients* 11, 2 (2019): 333.

104. Z. Qiao et al. *Schisandra chinensis* acidic polysaccharide improves the insulin resistance in type 2 diabetic rats by inhibiting inflammation. *J Med Food* 23, 4 (2020): 358–366.

105. M. Zhangu et al. *Schisandra chinensis* fructus and its active ingredients as promising resources for the treatment of neurological diseases. *Int J Mol Sci.* 19, 7 (2018): 1970.

106. A. McIntyre & M. Boudin. *Dispensing with Tradition: A Practitioner's Guide to Using Indian and Western Herbs the Ayurvedic Way* (2012).

107. S. Lianlin et al. The anti-colitis effect of *Schisandra chinensis* polysaccharide is associated with the regulation of the composition and metabolism of gut microbiota. *Frontiers Cell Infect Microbiol.* 10 (2020): 541.

108. S.B. Yoon et al. Anti-inflammatory effects of *Scutellaria*

baicalensis water extract on LPS-activated RAW 264.7 macrophages. *J Ethnopharmacol.* 125, 2 (2009): 286–290.

109. H. Liao et al. The main bioactive compounds of *Scutellaria baicalensis* Georgi. for alleviation of inflammatory cytokines: a comprehensive review. *Biomed Pharmacother.* 133 (2021): 110917.

110. H. Na et al. *Scutellaria baicalensis* alleviates insulin resistance in diet-induced obese mice by modulating inflammation. *Int J Mol Sci.* 20, 3 (2019): 727.

111. A. McIntyre & M. Boudin. *Dispensing with Tradition: A Practitioner's Guide to Using Indian and Western Herbs the Ayurvedic Way* (2012).

112. M. Bahmani et al. *Silybum marianum*: beyond hepatoprotection. *J Evid Based Complementary Altern Med.* 20, 4 (2015): 292–301.

113. C.M. Uritu et al. Medicinal plants of the family Lamiaceae in pain therapy: a review. *Pain Res Manag.* 2018 (2018): 7801543.

114. A.L. Araújo et al. In vivo wound healing effects of *Symphytum officinale* L. leaves extract in different topical formulations. *Pharmazie* 67, 4 (2012): 355–360.

115. F.E. Wirngo et al. The physiological effects of dandelion (*Taraxacum officinale*) in type 2 diabetes. *Rev Diabetic Stud.* 13, 2–3 (2016): 113–131.

116. S.M. Patil et al. A systematic review on ethnopharmacology, phytochemistry and pharmacological aspects of *Thymus vulgaris* Linn. *Heliyon* 7, 5 (2021): e07054.

117. M. Wood. *The Earthwise Herbal*, vol. 1: *A Complete Guide to Old World Medicinal Plants* (2008).

118. A. McIntyre & M. Boudin. *Dispensing with Tradition: A Practitioner's Guide to Using Indian and Western Herbs the Ayurvedic Way* (2012).

119. C. Hobbs. *Medicinal Mushrooms, the Essential Guide* (2020).

120. S.G. Lee et al. Anti-inflammatory and antioxidant effects of anthocyanins of *Trifolium pratense* (red clover) in lipopolysaccharide-stimulated RAW-267.4 macrophages. *Nutrients* 12, 4 (2020): 1089.

121. L. Krenn et al. Inhibition of angiogenesis and inflammation by an extract of red clover (*Trifolium pratense* L.). *Phytomedicine* 16, 12 (2009): 1083–1088.

122. M. Khazaei et al. Antiproliferative effect of *Trifolium pratense* L. extract in human breast cancer cells. *Nutr Cancer* 71, 1 (2019): 128–140.

123. N. Neelakantan et al. Effect of fenugreek (*Trigonella foenum-graecum* L.) intake on glycemia: a meta-analysis of clinical trials. *Nutr J* 13 (2014): 7.

124. A.S. Rao et al. *Nigella sativa* and *Trigonella foenum-graecum* supplemented chapatis safely improve HbA1c, body weight, waist circumference, blood lipids, and fatty liver in overweight and diabetic subjects: a twelve-week safety and efficacy study. *J Med Food* 23, 9 (2020): 905–919.

125. K. Spelman et al. Modulation of cytokine expression by traditional medicines: A review of herbal immunomodulators. *Altern Med Rev.* 11, 2 (2006): 128–150.

126. A. Serrano et al. Bioactive compounds and extracts from traditional herbs and their potential anti-inflammatory health effects. *Medicines* (Basel, Switzerland) 5, 3 (2018): 76.

127. A. Jacquet et al. Phytalgic, a food supplement, vs placebo in patients with osteoarthritis of the knee or hip: a randomised double-blind placebo-controlled clinical trial. *Arthritis Res Ther.* 11, 6 (2009): R192.

128. A.U. Turker et al. Common mullein (*Verbascum thapsus* L.): recent advances in research. *Phytother Res.* 19, 9 (2005): 733–739.

129. G. Calabrese et al. Phytochemical analysis and anti-inflammatory and anti-osteoarthritic bioactive potential of *Verbascum thapsus* L. (Scrophulariaceae) leaf extract evaluated in two in vitro models of inflammation and osteoarthritis. *Molecules* 26, 17 (2021): 5392.

130. M.A. Panchal. Pharmacological properties of *Verbascum thapsus* – a review. *Int J Pharma Sci Rev & Res.* 5, 2 (2010): Article-015.

131. M. Evans et al. Cancer patients' experiences of using mistletoe (*Viscum album*): a qualitative systematic review and synthesis. *J Altern Complement Med.* 22, 2 (2016): 134–144.

132. P. Hegde et al. *Viscum album* exerts anti-inflammatory effect by selectively inhibiting cytokine-induced expression of cyclooxygenase-2. *PLoS One* 6, 10 (2011): e26312.

133. M. Gupta et al. *Withania somnifera* (L.) Dunal ameliorates neurodegeneration and cognitive impairments associated with systemic inflammation. *BMC Complement Altern Med.* 19, 1 (2019): 217.

134. L.C. Mishra et al. Scientific basis for the therapeutic use of *Withania somnifera* (ashwagandha): a review. *Altern Med Rev.* 5, 4 (2000): 334–346.

135. R. Terry et al. The use of ginger (*Zingiber officinale*) for the treatment of pain: a systematic review of clinical trials. *Pain Med.* 12, 12 (2011): 1808–1018.

136. N.S. Mashhadi et al. Anti-oxidative and anti-inflammatory effects of ginger in health and physical activity: review of current evidence. *Int J Preventive Med.* 4, Suppl 1 (2013): S36–S42.

Resources

Finding a herbal practitioner in the UK and Ireland
These professional organisations all have a 'find a herbalist' page on their websites:

- Association of Master Herbalists (AMH) https://associationofmasterherbalists.co.uk
- College of Practitioners of Phytotherapy (CPP) https://thecpp.uk
- International Register of Consultant Herbalists and Homeopaths (IRCH) http://irch.org
- Irish Association of Master Medical Herbalists https://iammh.com
- Irish Register of Herbalists https://irh.ie
- National Institute of Medical Herbalists (NIMH) https://nimh.org.uk
- United Register of Herbal Practitioners (URHP) https://www.urhp.com

The Herb Society https://herbsociety.org.uk/

Recommended herbal suppliers who will supply to non-professional herbalists

- G. Baldwin and Co. https://www.baldwins.co.uk
- Neals Yard Remedies https://www.nealsyardremedies.com
- Tree Harvest https://www.tree-harvest.com

Herbal plant and seed suppliers
There are very many of these, and this is just a selection:

- British Wild Flower plants https://www.wildflowers.co.uk
- Herbal Haven https://www.herbalhaven.com
- Hooks Green Herbs https://www.hooksgreenherbs.com
- Norfolk Herb Nursery https://www.norfolkherbs.co.uk
- Poyntzfield Herb Nursery https://www.poyntzfieldherbs.co.uk
- The Herb Nursery https://www.herbnursery.co.uk

Essential oil suppliers.
These also need care with choice as there are some cheap and not very good essential oils out there. If it is cheap, it may not be good-quality.

These I know are good, but there may well be others I don't know.

- Fragrant Earth Organics https://www.fragrantearth.com
- Oshadhi https://oshadhi.co.uk
- Essential oils online https://www.essentialoilsonline.co.uk

Flower remedies
Bach Flower Remedies https://www.bachremedies.com
The Bach remedies are also available at many other outlets, both online and shop.

These companies sell Bach essences plus many other different essence ranges too and can all be recommended:

- International Flower Essence Repertoire https://www.healingorchids.com
- Crystal Herbs https://www.crystalherbs.com
- Saskia's Flower Essences https://www.saskiasfloweressences.com/

Supplements
These are freely available online and in many high street chemists and health food shops.

Index

Bold type indicates a main entry

B

B cells 15, 27

bacterial endotoxin 35

Baptisia tinctoria 30, 70, 71, **160–1**

barberry: see *Berberis vulgaris*

Barosma betulina 145, **161**

Bellis perennis 146, 159, **161**

Berberis vulgaris 22, 23, 33, 81, 144, 146, 148, **162**

bile acids 31, 68

black pepper: see *Piper nigrum*

bladder 9, 12, 22, 54, 75–8, 81, 84–5, 155, 156, 159, 161, 172, 173, 175, 196, 198, 205

Blautia obeum 38

blessed thistle: see *Carbenia benedicta*

bone broth 36, 120–1, 129

boneset: see *Eupatorium perfoliatum*

Boswellia serrata 20,22, 23, 109, **162–3**

bowels, function 23, 68, 69, 70, 162, 165, 193–4

    irritated 19, 75, 90, 93

bradykinin 14

bronchiectasis 98–9

bronchitis 98, 158, 175, 201

buchu: see *Barosma betulina*

burdock: see *Arctium lappa*

C

Calendula officinalis 20, 30, 33, 36, 81, **163**

cancer 9, 12, 27, 28, 38, 44, 50, 58, 66, 86, 108–9, 115, 119, 135, 143, 154, 155, 163, 164, 179, 180, 194, 195, 196, 197, 201, 202, 203, 205

Cannabis sativa, C. indica 109, **163–4**

capillary permeability 14, 143

Capsicum annuum 144, 145, **164**

Carbenia benedicta 33, 37, 97, 144, **165–6**

cardamom: see *Elettaria cardamomum*

cardiovascular disease 9, 12, 19, 38, 44, 47, 50, 58, 60, 62, 65, 66, 86–7, 115, 116–18, 133, 134, 137, 139, 140, 141, 144, 147, 160, 162, 164, 167, 168, 175, 177, 186, 194, 197

cat's claw: see *Uncaria tomentosa*

cayenne: see *Capsicum annuum*

celery seed: see *Apium graveolens*

Centaurium erythraea 37, 78, **166**

centaury: see *Centaurium erythraea*

Centella asiatica 80, 103, 148, **166**

chamomile: see *Matricaria chamomilla* and *Anthemis nobilis*

Chionanthus virginicus 33, 70, **167**

cholestasis 31

cholesterol 19, 31, 52, 55, 87, 116, 131, 134, 168, 170, 179, 187, 199, 201

chronic fatigue 9, 12, 63–4, 65, 80, 87–8, 89, 109, 176, 182, 202, 203

Cinnamomum spp. 112, 113, 127, 128, 129, 144, 150, 158, **167**

cinnamon: see *Cinnamomum spp.*

circulatory system 68, 71, 154, 164, 167, 168, 172, 176, 177, 193, 196, 204

cleavers: see *Galium aparine*

coeliac disease 42, 79, 113

comfrey: see *Symphytum officinale*

coriander: see *Coriandrum sativum*

Coriandrum sativum 37, 101, 120, 121, 127, 168

corn silk: see *Zea mays*

Corydalis spp. 109, 128, **168**

couch grass root: see *Agropyron repens*

COVID 39, 47, 58, 65, 87, 92, 135, 195

Crataegus oxyacantha 48, 87, 100, 130, 146, 149, 158, **168**

C reactive protein (CRP) 19, 92, 134, 135, 136, 138, 142

Crohn's disease 95

Inflammation

Juglans nigra 30, 40, 82, 116, 127, **183**

K

kidney(s) 20, 31, 42, 43, 47, 58, 66, 68, 69, 70, 141, 154, 156, 158, 159, 160, 161, 165, 169, 172, 173, 175, 179, 190, 198, 199

L

L-glutamine 76, 96–7
lack of exercise 47, 51, 61–2
leaky gut 34, 36, 40, 65, 113
lectins 54, **114**
lemon balm: see *Melissa officinalis*
Leonurus cardiaca 21, 100, **183**
linden: see *Tilia europaeus*
linseed: see *Linum usitatissimum*
Linum usitatissimum 40, 89, 93, 149, **185**
lipopolysaccharide (LPS) 35, 61, 105, 156, 158, 172, 173
lipoxygenase (LOX) 15, 158
liquorice: see *Glycyrrhiza glabra*
liver 19, 20, 23, 30–3, 35, 37, 42, 43, 63, 65, 68, 69, 70, 75, 81, 82, 89, 92, 103, 109, 135, 136, 141, 153–4, 155, 156, 158, 159, 160, 161, 162, 163, 164, 165–6, 167, 169, 170, 173, 175, 179, 180, 183, 186, 193–4, 195, 196, 197, 198–9, 201, 203, 206
Lobelia inflata 56, 64, 99, 101, **185–6**
lupus 66, 79, 80, 108, 139
Lycopus europaeus 21, **186**
lymph/lymphatic 23, 30, 70, 80, 81, 103, 144, 160, 163, 170, 175, 183, 190, 193, 196, 201, 202, 203
lymphocytes 14, 15, 27, 98, 134

M

magnesium 21, 63, 76, 89, 97, 123, 133, **136–8**
Mahonia aquifolium 63, 70, 71, 103,

148, **186**
maitake: see *Grifola frondosa*
marigold: see *Calendula officinalis*
Marrubium vulgare **186**
marshmallow: see *Althaea officinalis*
mast cells 14
Matricaria chamomilla 113, 127, 128, 149, **187**
meditation 45, 139–41, 178
Melissa officinalis 21, 46, 127, 130, 149, **187–8**
mental health 9, 12, 21, 61, 107–8, 198
Mentha piperita 90, 144, 145, **188**
mercury 66
metabolic disease/syndrome 17, 49, 60–2, 68, 91–3, 111, 119, 131, 139, 141, 158, 162, 164, 167, 179, 188, 194, 201, 202
microbiome
gut 9, 29, 30, 31, 35, 36, 38–41, 62, 66, 73, 74, 76, 102, 105, 107, 108, 113, 201
mouth 64
milk thistle: see *Silybum marianum*
mistletoe: see *Viscum album*
molecular mimicry 79, 112–13
motherwort: see *Leonurus cardiaca*
mugwort: see *Artemisia vulgaris*
mullein: see *Verbascum thapsus*
multiple sclerosis 17, 113

N

neem: see *Azadirachta indica*
nervous system 21, 28, 30, 42–6, 61, 66, 105, 116, 137, 145, 155, 165, 166, 168, 170, 177, 179, 181, 185, 187, 197, 200, 203, 204, 206, 207
nettle: see *Urtica dioica*
neurodegenerative disease 9, 12, 35, 66, 104–6, 159, 164, 195, 204
neuroinflammation 105–6, 166, 178, 191, 193

neutrophils 14, 15
nightshade intolerance 23, 54, 58, 80, 112, 114, **124–5**
nitric oxide 35, 47, 98, 173, 185
non steroidal anti inflammatory drugs (NSAIDs) 80–1, 141, 148

O

obesity 35, 47, 51, 52, 60–1, 65, 73, 79, 91, 92, 135, 141, 167, 195
Ocimum sanctum 23, 56, 99, 101, 148, **188**
oils and fats 31, 52, 111, 116–18
omega 3,6 fatty acids 27, 46, 49, 52, 116–18, 139
orange, bitter 37, **167**
Oregon grape root: see *Mahonia aquifolium*
osteoarthritis 21, 44, 55, 77, 93, 139, 148, 202
osteoporosis 9,12, 108, 136

P

Panax ginseng 30, 147, 149, **190, 204**
Parkinson's disease 104, 166
pectin 36
peppermint: see *Mentha piperita*
periodontal disease 79, 92, 95
periodontitis 51, 58, 64–5, 105, 172
phagocytes 14, 26, 134, 137
Phytolacca decandra 70, 144, **190**
phytonutrients 111, 114–15
Pimpinella anisum 53, 92, 122, 173, **190**
Piper nigrum 20, 37, 47, 53, 94, 145, 169, **190**
Plantago lanceolata and *P. major* 36, 53, 54, 63, 130, 149, **191**
plantain: see *Plantago lanceolata* and *P. major*
platelets 16, 47, 98
poke: see *Phytolacca decandra*
Polygonum cuspidatum 148, **191**
Porphyromonas gingivalis 106, 172

prebiotics 40–1, 96, 201
prickly ash: see *Zanthoxylum spp.*
probiotics 40–1, 44, 63, 76, 78, 82, 94, 99, 108, 122
prostaglandins 14, 15
Prunella vulgaris 56, **191–3**
psoriasis 40, 102, 163
psychoneuroimmunology 28, 61

R

red clover: see *Trifolium pratense*
reishi: see *Ganoderma lucidum*
rheumatoid arthritis 17, 20, 25, 66, 77, 79, 108, 113, 134, 139, 202
Rhodiola rosea 46, 148, **193**
Rosa canina 48, 127–8, 147, **193**
rose: see *Rosa canina*
rosemary: see *Salvia rosmarinus*
roseroot: see *Rhodiola rosea*
Rumex crispus 23, 33, 63, 70, 71, 81, 144, **193–4**

S

sage: see *Salvia officinalis*
sage, red: see *Salvia miltiorrhiza*
salicylate 54, 55, 58, 75, 76, 78, 82–3, 84, 88, 90, 93, 96, 103, 112, 113, **125–8**, 167, 169, 188, 195
Salvia miltiorrhiza 48, **194**
Salvia officinalis 30, 127, **194**
Salvia rosmarinus 33, 71, 127, 144, 145, 148, **195**
sariva: see *Hemidesmus indicus*
sauna 29, 68
saw palmetto: see *Serenoa repens*
Schisandra chinensis 46, 128, **195–6**
Scrophularia nodosa 30, 63, 70, **196**
Scutellaria baicalensis 53, 75, 148, **196**
Scutellaria lateriflora 33, 46, **196–7**
secretory IgA 40
selenium 29, 133, **138–9**
selfheal: see *Prunella vulgaris*
Serenoa repens 147, **197**
serotonin 14

sex hormones 51, 59, 65
shatavari: see *Asparagus racemosus*
Silybum marianum 20, 33, 75, 82, 92, 149, 160, **197**
sinusitis 22–3, 58, 81, 99, 107, 158, 198
Sjogren's 76–7, 81–2
skullcap: see *Scutellaria lateriflora*
skullcap, Baical: see *Scutellaria baicalensis*
sleep 21, 22–3, 28, 39, 43–4, 51, 53, 54, 61, 81, 85, 88–90, 96, 100–1, 103-4, 107, 137, 156, 164, 168, 175, 187, 204, 206
slippery elm: see *Ulmus fulva*
smoking 47, 49, 51, 65, 98
Solidago virgaurea 64, 78, 100, 101, 146, **197–8**
soya intolerance 21, 54, 63, 76, 79, 101, 112, 123
Stachys betonica 85, 101, **198**
stimulant herbs 13, 32, 69, 70, 71, **143–4**
St John's wort: see *Hypericum perforatum*
stress 20, 28, 32, 39, 41–4, 51, 55, 61, 64, 79, 82, 87, 96, 100, 107, 124, 129, 131, 134, 138, 139, 140, 147, 156, 166, 173, 175, 181, 188, 194, 196, 200, 203, 204
stroke 66, 86, 116, 136, 139, 141, 195
sugar 17, 27, 30, 39, 47, 51–2, 107, 111, 120, 122, 127, 179
Symphytum officinale 55, **198**

T
T cells 15, 27, 31
Taraxacum officinale 23, 33, 69, 71, 81, 103, 130, 144, 149, 150, 158, **199**
thrombosis 47, 83, 86, 135, 137
Thymus vulgaris, T. mastichina 30, 99, 127, **200**
thyme: see *Thymus vulgaris, T. mastichina*

Tilia europaeus 46, 146, **200**
tonic herbs 22, 23, 30, 32, 37, 46, 56, 54, 69, 82, 87, 99, 100, 143, 145–7, 155, 159, 160, 172, 181, 188, 190, 194, 197, 199, 207
toxins, toxicity 51, 61, 66–8, 79, 98, 103, 124, 134, 141, 143, 158–9, 161, 173, 175, 194, 206
Trametes versicolor 14, 148, **200–1**
trans fats 17, 30, 35, 51–2, 111, 116
Trifolium pratense 70, 71, 80, **201**
Trigonella foenum-graecum 92, 94, 127, **201**
turkey tail: see *Trametes versicolor*
turmeric: see *Curcuma longa*

U
ulcerative colitis 95–7
urinary tract infection 58, 198; see also: cystitis
Ulmus fulva 36, 40, 93, 96–7, 149, **201**
Uncaria tomentosa 149, **201**
Urtica dioica 54, 69, 80, 92, 130, 147, 148, **202**

V
vagus nerve 42–6, 164, 166, 185, 187
vasoconstrictor 47
vasodilator 14, 47, 100, 153, 160, 200, 203
Verbascum thapsus 71, **202**
Verbena officinalis 33, 97, 103, **203**
vervain: see *Verbena officinalis*
Viola odorata 78, **203**
Viola tricolor 30, 103, 147, **203**
violet: see *Viola odorata, V. tricolor*
viral infection 14, 58, 65, 87, 93, 106, 113, 139, 173
Viscum album 100, **203–4**
vitamin A 115, 116, **133**
vitamin B 31, 40, 81, 129, **133**
vitamin C 29, 63, 76, 81, 89, 97, **134,** 193

vitamin D3 20, 29, 63, 76, 81, 89,
       116, 129, 133, **135**
vitamin E 116, 118, **136,** 202
vitamin K 116
vulnerary 23, 56, 64, 82, 93, 96, 99,
       101, 163, 198, 207

W
walnut: see *Juglans nigra*
white horehound: see *Marrubium*
       vulgare
wild indigo: see *Baptisia tinctoria*
wild yam: see *Dioscorea villosa*
Withania somnifera 22, 30, 46, 64,
       80, 82, 83, 89, 147, 149, **204**
wood betony: see *Stachys betonica*

Y
yarrow: see *Achillea millefolium*
yellow dock: see *Rumex crispus*
yerba mansa: see *Anemopsis*
       californica

Z
Zanthoxylum spp. 71, 144, **204**
Zea mays 76, 85, 154, **204–5**
zinc 29, 133, **138**
Zingiber officinale 13, 20, 23, 37, 47,
       48, 53, 71, 80, 82, 96, 97,
       120–1, 127, 144, 145, 148,
       187, **205**
zonulin 34

CPSIA information can be obtained
at www.ICGtesting.com
Printed in the USA
JSHW050811080922
30203JS00007B/8